Daughters

of

Divine Destiny

DEMETRIA LEBLANC

Best Wishes,
D. LeBlanc

Daughters of Divine Destiny:
A Good Sense Guide to Godly Womanhood

by Demetria LeBlanc

ISBN: 978-1-936497-23-2

Searchlight Press

Who are you looking for?

Publishers of thoughtful Christian books since 1994.

5634 Ledgestone Drive

Dallas, Texas 75214

info@Searchlight-Press.com

www.Searchlight-Press.com

www.JohnCunyus.com

This book is dedicated to the present
Daughters of Divine Destiny
and future generations to come, especially to the divine daughters in my life, to my grand-daughters, Brooklyn & Nyla. To my nieces; Ashlynn, Ava, Blake, Payton, Jasmine, Kennedy & Trinity

Table of Contents

Acknowledgement   i

Foreword   x

Introduction   xii

1 - Knowing Your Worth   1

2 - Respect   23

3 - Friendship   37

4 - Hygiene   48

5 - Dating/Relationships   62

6 - Sex (Parental Discretion is Advised, if under 18)   83

7 - Life Skills   106

8 - College/Career   129

9 - Your Salvation   141

10 - Words of Wisdom   151

References   158

Acknowledgements

Wow, what a journey this has been. Who would have thought all the emotions and reservations that had to be dealt with to get to the point of finishing this book? It has been a roller coaster ride of digging down deep inside of my inner being to uncover emotions and events that were buried a long time ago, only to be uncovered and dealt with for such a time as this.

I am ever so grateful for all my life experiences and the people who have shared them with me, to presently be at a place of wholeness to help others get to where I am today; a life full of love, peace, and blessings. This journey wasn't easy for me, but I hope and pray my transparency was worth it to help God's Daughters get to their place of destiny.

I would like to give thanks to the wonderful women in my life that have helped shape me on my journey. First, to my wonderful Mama, Rev. Linda

Ross, a true woman of God that exemplifies fierce determination, courage, character, and dignity in her life daily by being a true Proverbs 31 woman. My mother has always been a true, driving force in me succeeding in whatever I chose to do. I cherish you, Mama, for the foundation you instilled in me that has helped me to become a Godly woman, mother, and wife. I couldn't be half the woman I am today without your wonderful example. I love you always. To my wonderful grandmother, Vallie Campbell Rogers, who has always nurtured me as her own, given me Godly wisdom, been my rock, and fed me and my family good food (spiritual and physical) throughout the years. My grandmother was my sons' babysitter until they reached school age, which is why I have one son that's an old soul, and all three of them have God-filled, morally decent spirits. That wasn't by happenstance; it was a village that helped mold and shape them. Thanks, Mama *(I call my grandmother Mama, too)*, for always being there for me. I can never repay you for your love and kindness. You will always be in my heart; I love you!   To my mother-in–law, Audrey Hall, I couldn't ask for a better mother-in-law. She is my second Mama, whom I call Mom. Mom is that woman who makes sure everything is alright and that everybody has something. No one is left behind. She is a true giver. She has taught me so many things: how to cook that good Louisiana food, how to thrift shop and make a dollar stretch until it screams, how to manage my husband and my household, the list could go on and on. I want to thank you, Mom, for treating me as one of your daughters (not just a daughter-in-law) and loving me as true family. I love you! To the late, great Mrs. Rozelia Frank LeBlanc, Mawmaw, as we call her, was one of a kind. She didn't take no (any) mess and told you exactly what was on her mind. Mawmaw is my husband's grandmother and we grew awfully close when she left her home in Louisiana to come stay with my family, my husband Chris, Sr., my sons, Chris, Jr. (1 ½) and my newborn, Quincy, while I was in and out of the hospital from blood clots and other complications from child birth. I will forever be grateful to her for leaving her home in the country to come and see about us in the city. She didn't have to do it, but having a love for family and being an unselfish woman, she came for well over a month and cooked, cleaned, and took care of my babies while I got well. I'm so glad I expressed my gratitude to her while she was still alive.   Mawmaw, you will forever be in my heart; you took care of us when we needed you the most and you did it so lovingly. That's true family. I love and miss you dearly.

To the women I have grown into womanhood with, created history and shared enough love and laughter to last a lifetime. To Kimberly Palmer, my cousin/sister, thanks for making growing up without a sister bearable and always being that substitute. We have had so many cherished moments growing up; hope to make more growing older. I love you. To my sisters-in-law, Antisher Ben, Antionette Hood (Netta), and Angela Green (Ann), I must say you all have truly given me the experience of what it means to have sisters - the good, the bad and the ugly of it. You all are the cream of the crop. Just thinking about the times we have shared makes me want to laugh and cry, all at the same time. Thanks for always being there as true sisters; y'all are the very best. I love you all. To my besties, Nolotta LeBlanc and Christie Jones, thanks for being a good friend. I know I can talk to y'all daily or not for weeks at a time and it's all good. Thanks for being my sounding board to listen to my problems and complaints or another bright idea. You all are the best. I love you! To my late best friend, the beautiful Reshanda Williams, gone too soon, who died at the early age of 36, I miss you and will keep our legacy of reaching out to young women alive in your honor; I love you and miss you always. To Reshanda's mother, Mama Lillian Williams, my Titus 2 mentor, thanks for all the wisdom, encouragement, and knowledge you poured into me. I will always remember us sitting on your porch in silence as I pondered one of my biggest life decisions while you waited patiently for my answer to your question – "What do you want to do?" I love you and cherish the times we have shared. To my daughter-in-law (my very first girl), Leeandra LeBlanc, who I love as my very own daughter, I couldn't have prayed for a better wife for my son. Thanks for loving my son the way you do and being his Proverbs 31 wife. You have brought so much joy and excitement into all of our lives; I love you. To the mother of my grandchildren, (Jaedon, Brooklyn & Christian), Laketria Brumfield, thanks for allowing me to pour into your life as I would my very own daughter. I believe God placed you in my life so I could have a first-hand experience of what it's like for a young woman today trying to maneuver into womanhood and motherhood, all at the same time. I love you and will always be there for you. To the mother of my grand-daughter Nyla, Shenequa Emerson, thank you for your kind sweet spirit and taking such good care of my grandbaby. I love and cherish you for it.

To all the wonderful women that have come across my path for one reason or another, especially the C&M Strong Ministries (Aunt Mae), thank you for all the influence, encouragement and spiritual growth you have brought to my life. I can't name all of you, but know you are appreciated.

To my Pastor, Dr. David Henderson, Jr. and First Lady, Dr. Kathy Henderson, thanks for all the spiritual guidance, teachings, and training that has kept me spiritually grounded. I love you. You all are the best!

To my awesome grandfather, NB Rogers, thanks for being the epitome of a good, God-fearing man and providing us with love and wisdom. You take such good care of my grandmother and I love you for it.

To my amazing brothers and sister-in-law, Rev. Solomon Evans and Sedrick & Kim Evans, thanks for being such a wonderful part of my life. Solomon, thanks for showing me how God can work through people to get the very best out of them. Your life is a living testimony of that very fact. Keep preaching the uncompromising Word. I love you. Sedrick, my baby brother, you have such a sweet spirit and are a man of honor. I love you and cherish our relationship. I hope and pray you get to feel God's presence one day soon; you'll never be the same again. Kim, thanks for being a good, loving, kind, and sweet person. You have a heart for family and I love you for it.

To my three handsome sons, Christopher LeBlanc, Jr., Quincy LeBlanc, and Malcolm LeBlanc, my life's treasure to the world. I love and appreciate you all more than you could ever know. I couldn't have asked for better children. It has been such a joy raising you all. Raising God-fearing, respectable, intelligent, independent, and honorable young men was our purpose and, I must say, you all have exceeded our expectations; to God be all the glory.

Last, but most certainly not least, to my wonderful, wonderful husband, Christopher LeBlanc, Sr. I never thought at the young age of seventeen I would meet my nineteen year old soul mate and we would share a lifetime of emotions, events, situations, setbacks, and blessings. You have brought so much joy and happiness to my life throughout the years. You are the greatest husband, father, and friend. The road hasn't been easy, but it sure has been worth it and I cherish each day as we grow older together and enjoy the fruits of our labor through our sons and their families.

God Is Good All The Time, And All The Time, God Is Good!

Foreword

I was delighted when my good friend, Demetria LeBlanc, asked me to write the foreword to her book, <u>Daughters of Divine Destiny</u>. This book exemplifies **ministry in action**. In an increasingly secular environment, Demetria saw the need for young women to have a practical guide which not only would give them hope, but also help in life's difficult situations.

As a young woman, Demetria knows firsthand the importance of putting first things first. She quickly learned that not only did God have a plan for her life, but so did Satan. It was through her many challenging circumstances and trying times she learned that God had to be the foundation of her life. I have seen her passion and desire to help young women who are married and maybe miserable, or single and dissatisfied, realize their worth.

Demetria has taken Paul's epistle to Titus seriously (Titus 2:3), and turned it into a step by step approach for young women to make better choices that will produce a positive outcome. She follows Christ's example showing the need for Christians to stoop down in order to lift up those who are downcast. Demetria sees the fruit on the vines which are ready for harvesting, and her question is, "Where are the laborers?"

I feel you will be blessed and benefited by this book in a remarkable way. My prayer for you is that you will open up your heart to receive this important message.

Dr. Kathy Harris Henderson
Dallas, Texas

Introduction

"Teach Them the Way They Should Go"

³ Likewise, teach the older women to be reverent in the way they live, not to be slanderers or addicted to much wine, but to teach what is good.⁴ Then they can urge the younger women to love their husbands and children, ⁵ to be self-controlled and pure, to be busy at home, to be kind, and to be subject to their husbands, so that no one will malign the word of God. *Titus 2:3-5 (NIV)*

"Daughters of Divine Destiny" is a *Good Sense Guide to Godly Womanhood* that shares Godly principles on life values that every young woman needs to know and have to become a *Daughter of Divine Destiny*. We all start out in life ignorant of what to do, how to do, when to do or where to do the most important fundamentals of life. Most of us are born into families where we are taught their values and ways of life. Our family's way of life shapes us into the person we will ultimately become. However, we have become a society that is so obsessed with materialism and worldly standards that we have neglected to teach and raise up a generation of self-respecting, young women. Because of this neglect, we have become an "anything goes" society and we do as the world dictates. This mentality has caused a lost generation that is producing children at an alarming rate to create an even more lost generation. Somehow, some way, we have to take a stand and reach out to help those that are lost by telling our story, to help them have an even better story. We need to stop and share with them the basic knowledge of life, of how to become morally productive, God-fearing, young women so they're not left wondering what, when, where, why, or how to do the most important fundamentals of life.

We have forgotten about the precious pearls that are being left behind to fend for themselves; the young ladies, be it a family member or our own children. They are left behind for material or selfish gains. Traditional values *(we don't talk about that)* or ignored and neglected for one reason or another, and they are given trinkets, if anything at all, to compensate for the guilt that is felt for the quality time not spent to love and nurture them. So often, young women get information from all the wrong places, i.e. music videos/lyrics, television, friends, the internet, etc. They are filled with so much wrong information that they are transformed into these artificial beings becoming products of their environments that are structured in chaos.

"Daughters of Divine Destiny" is a Godly instructed guide written to fill in the cracks of today's life knowledge that is left unfilled or misguided. It's a guide for young women to live by and strive towards.

Hosea 4:6 NIV

My people are destroyed from lack of knowledge...

This guide contains very sensitive and straightforward information to decrease confusion, to reveal knowledge and wisdom that can be used for better decision making.

one

KNOWING
YOUR WORTH

"Show Your Worth, So Others Will Know Your Worth"

[13] For you created my inmost being; you knit me together in my mother's womb.[14] I praise you because I am fearfully and wonderfully made; your works are wonderful, I know that full well. *Psalm 139:13-14 (NIV)*

Dear Divine Daughter,

Self-Worth (value of self) starts with loving yourself. You have to love yourself to know you're worthy of respect, first from yourself and then from others.

> Nobody should treat you better/worse than you treat yourself.

Not knowing your worth is a huge concern. God said you were fearfully (powerfully) and wonderfully (perfectly) made. He loved you so much that He made you an extraordinary being, not just ordinary. You are a one of a kind creation; there's not another person like you. He knitted your most intricate parts in your mother's womb, making you a unique person. But if you don't know your worth (which is priceless, by the way), you will look for validation of your worth in all the wrong things and people, sometimes even using your body seductively to receive validation of worth from men. Let me tell you, you are loved more than you will ever know, first, by God the Father (who sent His son Jesus to die for your sins), second, by Jesus the son (who died for your sins), and third, by saints that love the Lord and have a passion for young women to be whole and become the precious *Daughters of Divine Destiny* God created you to be.

Short Story: *Growing up I had very low self-esteem and did not love myself. Looking back I know it stemmed from not having a father in my* *life, feelings of not fitting in because I didn't have the latest fashions or devices, and most of all, not knowing God the way I do now. Growing up I felt unworthy because I was abandoned by my biological father (even though I had a loving mother); I missed that validation from my father, of what he thought of me as a daughter, and having his love, protection, and financial support. I never knew the feeling of calling someone Daddy or being Daddy's little girl. I grew up feeling that my Dad didn't love me, because if he did, he wouldn't have left me in this cold and cruel world to fend for myself without his support, never caring whether the seed he produced needed anything or was alright. I felt worthless because he wasn't there to love me. Don't get me wrong, I had a good upbringing because I had a good, loving, determined, and God-fearing mother that provided for me and my brothers. Living with a single parent, monetary resources were few, so I didn't have the latest fashions or devices. My needs were provided for, but the name brands and latest anything was not a part of my life. As a teen, you don't understand that those material things are not important. You feel that in order to fit in and feel valuable you need to have what everybody else has, and if you don't have it, you feel devalued. At least that's how I felt; I felt inferior to others who had what I didn't. I felt they were better than me, and I defined my worth based on that.*

In actuality, my worth was not defined by any of those things and neither is yours. I learned that I've always had a loving father protecting and providing for me. My Heavenly Father has never left me or rejected me, and when I realized that truth, I respected my worth as a person based on what my Heavenly Father says about me. You see, anybody can gain possession of material things (you have the money, you can buy it), but God gives you something that cannot be purchased. He gives you assets that can only come from within. Until you know this and tap into them, you will never truly know your worth. I tapped into mine and found my worth in Him, not man or material things.

As I stated before, *and can't stress enough*, you have to first love yourself – no matter your circumstances, then you have to respect yourself for who God created you to be. I know many of you don't love or respect yourselves because you don't know your worth. You feel you are unworthy because of not having a parent present, social status *(not having enough of this or that)*, looks, weight *(be it fat or skinny)*, skin color *(dark or light)*, hair texture, or any of those unique features that make you an original creation. Don't let anyone or anything define your worth; you define it by God's Word.

> You have to love and respect who God created you to be; to be a Godly young woman of worth whether someone likes you or not. If you're not confident in whom you are in Christ, you will let others demean you because of the lack of value you have placed on yourself.

In order to know what God says about you, you have to know who you are in Christ and have self-security, to know you're worth more than any of the latest devices or styles and name brands you wear *(that the world encourages you to buy to express a certain social status).* You're more than a pretty face that fades with time *(no amount of plastic surgery will stop it)* or a sexy body *(it's good to be healthy/fit but your body doesn't define your worth).* You need to know your worth is not based on anything physical; it's all spiritual. To know your self-worth, you need to know what God says and get your validation from Him instead of from any man, woman, magazine, or television commercial. Proverbs 31 describes a woman's worth. **A good woman is worth far more than rubies.** *(Proverbs 31:10)* **She is:**

- Trustworthy *(not deceitful, manipulative, or scheming),* **Proverbs 31:11**

- Nice *(not spiteful, mean, cruel, or hurtful),* **Proverbs, 31:12**

- A hard worker. She puts forth her best effort in everything she does, **Proverbs 31:13, 17-19**

- Resourceful with money, time, and talent – looks for ways to put them to good use, **Proverbs 31:14-16**

- Benevolent *(giving, compassionate, kind, caring - not selfish)*, **Proverbs 31:20**

- Organized and prepared, **Proverbs 31:21**

- Graceful *(well-groomed with whatever fashion she wears – name brands don't make her)*, **Proverbs 31:22**

- Respectable *(to self and others)*, **Proverbs 31:23**

- Goal oriented and business minded, **Proverbs 31:24**

- Of good character, **Proverbs 31:25**

- Wise *(gives Godly wisdom and does not gossip)*, **Proverbs 31:26**

- Efficient in her duties *(not lazy)* and clean *(neat and orderly)*, **Proverbs 31:27**

- Inspirational, motivational, and encouraging to others, **Proverbs 31:28-29**

- A Believer in God, a God-Filled Spirit, **Proverbs 31:30**

- Honorable and Praiseworthy, **Proverbs 31:31**

You have to focus on your inner beauty *(personality, attitude, and integrity)*, and have self-assurance in who you are as a person *(not anyone else's assurance)* which will ultimately transcend into confidence, personal appeal *(based off your inner being – that is eternal- it does not diminish)*, and self-respect. Taking care of your inner being will make you the most beautiful person on the outside because the <u>*divine authentic you*</u> will be on display, showing you are a woman of worth.

Now, don't confuse having confidence and self-respect with being stuck-up. You can feel good about yourself without thinking you are better than someone else or that someone is beneath you. Being respectful of yourself and having confidence in your self-worth is about knowing who you are in Christ and respecting others for who they are and will become.

THE WORTH OF YOUR BODY

¹⁹ Do you not know that your bodies are temples of the Holy Spirit, who is in you, whom you have received from God? You are not your own; *1 Corinthians 6:19 - NIV*

When my two oldest sons joined the US Military *(one the Air Force, the other the Army National Guard Reserves),* upon their completion of boot camp graduation, we all sat down to discuss their experiences. One thing in particular they told me that struck me as strange then, but has become clearer to me now, was when they said they were told, *"You are now the* **property** *of the United States Military."* I said "They view you all as property?" They said, "Yes, the property of the United States Military and we're responsible for taking care of their property, which is our bodies." Case in point, one comrade got into an altercation with another comrade and received a black eye. The US Military brought them up on charges for destroying military property; their bodies.

Just as they are the property of the United States Military until they finish their term, we, as believers, are the property of God and are responsible for taking care of His property (our bodies) until we die.

You are not your own; you were brought with a price, and when you go out into the world you represent our Heavenly Father. Divine Daughter, there are so many things to warn you about so you can be properly prepared for life. I truly believe that people perish for lack of knowledge. That's why knowledge is power for you to make wise choices to live the abundant life God has for you. I want to address every area of life that can cause severe detour and devastation, because _when you know better, you should do better._ Let's talk about some things we can do to harm our bodies.

Drugs

One area I know takes you down the wrong path is drugs, whether it's legal _(prescribed – taking prescription or over-the counter pills for an_ *illness is different than taking pills to experience a high)* or illegal (non-prescribed). You have to be very careful not to put anything in your body that might cause mind altering or addictive behavior.

You cannot fill your body with drugs and harmful chemicals. Your body is a temple to be loved and cared for by you, so you should treat it as such – keeping it clean and free of trash of any kind. Smoking, snorting, popping pills, or injecting any kind of substance isn't good for you.

> I know you may think it can't happen to you, but it can and it will if you experiment with the wrong thing or person.

You need to keep your mind clear so you can make sound and wise choices. Having it fogged with drugs, including alcohol, is just asking for trouble. I know young people like experimenting, but experimentation can cost you, big time; it's better to learn from someone else's mistakes *(there are plenty of examples to learn from - you don't have to look far).*

I have seen many people my age get hooked on drugs that look 15-20 years older than me and have never accomplished anything worthwhile with their lives. I have never had a desire to do drugs, because I have seen them destroy countless lives, some being close relatives. Believe me, *drugs are not something you want to try out just to see how it feels, because you might never be the same again*. There are numerous stories about mothers and fathers becoming hooked on drugs to the point they sell their kids for sex or abandon them looking for that next fix. The drug epidemic has claimed many families and is still robbing the communities of them today. You need to treat your body right; it's the only one you will have and using drugs will only make it deteriorate faster. Just say NO; it's not worth it.

> Always remember, the choices you make today are the choices you will live with tomorrow.

For more information on drug abuse, visit: http://www.drugabuse.gov/drugs-abuse.

Molestation / Inappropriate Touching

(To force unwanted sexual attentions on somebody)

The world is <u>not</u> a nice place and people are <u>not</u> always who they seem to be. They can seem really nice, and then turn really mean and vulgar. You have to be very careful of how someone tries to occupy your personal space. If you have an uneasy feeling about someone being too close to you or touching you inappropriately on or near your private parts *(breast, vagina, or buttocks)*, you need to <u>get away</u> from this situation and share this information with a <u>trusted adult,</u> i.e. parents, grandparents, teacher, mentor, aunt/uncle, pastor, etc., so they can deal with the situation with the proper response.

There have been several instances in the news where young girls have been molested by caregivers, a relative *(male and female)*, close friends of the family, teachers, total strangers *(Facebook friends)*, and even parents – no one is off limits. God has given each of us a discerning spirit *(some call it the female intuition)* where you can just feel something is not right. You should always pay close attention to that feeling of discernment because it could save you someday. Never be such a trusting person that you put yourself in harm's way. Pay attention to how a person treats you. If someone offers you money or gifts for some sort of inappropriate, physical contact, <u>say no</u>, and tell a trusted adult. I can't stress enough how important it is for you to get help. If you are molested, you are a victim of crime. Your action *(doing the right thing and telling someone)* may prevent others from becoming victims.

Here are some other things to watch out for:

- If someone is always giving you compliments on your body or body parts.

- If someone tries to play a sexual game or wrestle/tussle with you by touching you intimately or on your private parts.

- If someone wants you to keep a secret of something inappropriate or intimate they have done with you.

- If someone tells you dirty jokes or tries to make you watch pornography (sexual explicit movies).

- If someone gives you a lot of unnecessary, unwanted, inappropriate attention and tells you "you're special."

Pay attention and beware of predators that try to steal your innocence. Remember, it's not your fault and you need to tell a trusted adult.

Suicidal Thoughts

Divine Daughter, life is not easy and can sometimes leave you feeling lonely in this world. You may have feelings as if no one cares or understands anything you are going through, or even cares about you. You may feel as if the problems you're facing will never go away, but will just get worse. At the time you are feeling your lowest, thoughts of suicide might enter your mind as a solution to solve it all. But know this;

it is a trick of the enemy, Satan, whose job is to steal, kill, and destroy. *John 10:10-NIV, "The thief comes only to steal and kill and destroy; I have come that they may have life, and have it to the full."* Satan wants to get you to a place where you want to take your own life; the life Jesus died to give you. Do not be deceived by Satan's trickery. God is only a prayer away and you can rest in the peace of His arms, knowing all things *(good and bad)* work for the good of those who love the Lord. *Romans 8:28 – NIV, "And we know that in all things God works for the good of those who love him, who have been called according to his purpose."* I'm not telling you something I have heard, but what I truly know. Everything in life changes; nothing stays the same and that includes your situation. If you feel you're at your absolute lowest and don't feel like going on, you need to encourage yourself that this situation will pass and everything heals with enough time. If you cannot encourage yourself, then talk to someone you trust with your feelings to give you the right advice and the encouragement you need *(a parent or grandparent, your pastor, favorite aunt/uncle, mentor, etc.)* to help you through this dark time in your life. I'm a living testimony that things are not always as bad as they seem and given enough time and prayer, all wounds can be healed. Remember nothing, absolutely, positively, nothing is too hard for God. Don't let Satan rob you of your life. God loves you so much and will work everything *(the good, the bad and the ugly)* out for your benefit. Be not deceived; this too shall pass.

Short Story: *I knew someone who had thoughts of suicide; she tried ending her life. She was in a bad place emotionally and felt all alone. She didn't feel as if anyone cared about what she was going through or could even understand, nor did she tell anyone how she felt. <u>You see, secrecy is how Satan gets you alone in the darkness of your mind where you hide your true feelings from the world; you put on a mask to meet everyone's expectations, but deep, down inside you're hurting and no one knows it but you, Satan, and God.</u> She felt that her fate in life was ultimately* *to feel depressed and unloved. She didn't want to live like that and wanted the peace of not having to deal with any hurt, pain, or feelings of rejection anymore. She listened to a thought that was telling her it would all be better if she wasn't here. You have to realize Satan plants negative, evil, and destructive thoughts in your mind and comes to you when you're the most vulnerable, and usually that's when you're young, naïve, and ignorant of God's promises in His Word, plans for your life, and capabilities of His Power. In other words, he wants to get you when you don't know any better. So many young lives have been changed drastically early on because they just didn't know the tricks of the enemy. As for this young woman, she heard the Word, but she didn't know the Word. She didn't know how to apply it to her life or her situation. So the enemy tried to take her out, but GOD! At her lowest point, at the age of sixteen, she took a bottle of pills and waited for death to come. While waiting for death, she told people goodbye. They soon realized something was wrong and that she needed help. She was rushed to the hospital where she had to drink a black charcoal medicine to get the pills out of her system so no permanent damage would be done to her organs. After a day or so in the hospital, she had to speak to a psychiatrist so they could evaluate what had gotten her to that point so she wouldn't get there again. Honestly, she said the whole episode seemed like a bad dream. It was all a fog in her mind as to how she got to that place. In hindsight, it was like she was in a trance; just moving without thinking.*

Truly I tell you, if Satan's plan had worked, I wouldn't have the abundant life I have today to be able to tell you God has a plan and provision for all of our lives, and the struggles and situations we go through only make us stronger, to be able to help someone else along the way. I have gone through a lot of things in my life and felt, why me? But now I know it was for such a time as this; to be able to help God's daughters get to their divine destiny. So, you see, Satan tries to take you out before God's purpose for your life can be fulfilled. That's why you have to hold on to God's unchanging hand because he will never leave you nor forsake you. God is not a man that He should lie. Trust and believe He can and will turn your situation around. I sometimes think about that sixteen year old girl and wonder, if she wasn't here, who would have done my part? You know, we all have a part to play in the grand scheme of life. **<u>Don't let Satan rob you of your leading role.</u>**

Questions/Reflections

1) Where does self-worth start?

_____
_____
_____

2) From whom should you get your validation of worth?

_____
_____
_____

3) What are some things that might cause lack of self-worth?

_____
_____
_____

4) What are some characteristics of self-worth?

_____
_____
_____

5) What kind of drugs can harm your body?

_____
_____
_____

6) What are some signs of inappropriate
   touching/behavior?

_____
_____
_____

7) Who are sexual predators?

_____
_____
_____

8) When does Satan try to take you out?

_____
_____
_____

9) Self-Reflection: Do you love yourself?
   How will you become more like the Proverbs
   31 woman?

_____
_____
_____

two

RESPECT

Plant Good Seeds; Give Out What You Would Like In Return

So in everything, do to others what you would have them do to you, *Matthew 7:12 - NIV*

Dear Divine Daughter,

God's hopes and dreams for you as a young woman are endless and you can achieve much of what you want in life by always putting Him first and having the attribute of respect. *Matt 6:33-KJV, "But seek ye first the kingdom of God, and his righteousness; and all these things shall be added unto you."*

Respect is one of the single most important attributes you need to have, for yourself, your family, and those you encounter, to acquire the characteristics of being a Godly young woman. You need respect to obey God's rules, your parents' rules, society's rules and even rules/guidelines you set for yourself. To show respect, you have to know respect is reciprocated. You have to give it to get it and it goes in that order. You don't demand respect; it's given out to be given back in return.

As a respectable, Godly young woman you should always show respect, especially in these areas:

Respect of Your Elders – By addressing your elders with *Mr. or Ms.* and answering with a *Yes, Ma'am/No, Ma'am or Yes, Sir/No, Sir* shows the ultimate sign of respect. I remember growing up, my grandmother always told us to put a handle on it when addressing an adult or authority figure. By saying handle, we knew we better address them as Mr./Ms. or Aunt/Uncle or there was going to be trouble. I have found throughout the years that this single act of respect will carry you a long way in life, especially with those of influence *(teachers,* *officers, pastors, parents, etc.)* and they will respect you for it.

Respect the Use of Your Words – Many young women believe it's cool to use foul language because that's what they have seen others do. Growing up we felt the same way. We felt if we cursed it would make us feel grown up and cool. Little did we know we only looked foolish. I remember my cousin had just learned how to curse and she was firing them out her mouth one after the other; it wasn't making sense how she would use them. As she was firing them out, I thought to myself, she really looks silly. A Godly young woman speaks intelligently, without the need to use derogatory language to express herself, and she expresses herself without being offensive to those around her. A young woman also doesn't speak when she has nothing nice to say; it's not attractive for a young woman to tear someone down with hurtful words.

Respect of Your Conduct/Behavior – A Godly young woman carries herself with dignity *(self-worth)* and possesses decorum *(decency)* so people know she's about something *(a daughter of the most-high king, God)* and wants to be of value to society. She treats people the way she would like to be treated. I was taught the Golden Rule growing up: *"Do unto others **as you would have them** do unto you."* If you treat people right, you'll get treated right *(most of the time anyway, but you can only be responsible/ accountable for your actions, not theirs)*.

Respect of Your Appearance *(keep your body parts adequately covered, don't show all your assets – dress classy, not trashy)* – Fashions today leave little to the imagination as to what's beneath the clothes. As a young woman, you have to be careful not to dress inappropriately *(wearing tight-fitted pants; skirts, shorts, or dresses that barley cover your buttocks; low-cut shirts where everything is visible except the breast nipple)*; this labels you as sluttish and entices harmful attention from the opposite sex. *I call it hoochie-mama attention, because the boys think you're a good-time girl – just someone to have sex with. They will assume you're not worthy of dating* *because your appearance says you're not worth that type of quality time; that is reserved for girlfriend potential. Your appearance says you are not.* By revealing too much skin, <u>*you're sending a message*</u> that categorizes you as sexually loose *(anybody can have you);* even if that's not who you are, that's the message you're sending with your appearance. Please know this, if you dress like a prostitute, you will be identified and treated as one. The only difference they will see is *yours is free.* This is because you put yourself in the same category as the girls that have put themselves on the market to be used. You're not setting yourself apart to be something better than that *(a Divine Daughter)* or different from the rest, so you get treated the same.

Short Story:

Muhammad Ali's Advice To His Daughters:

An incident transpired when Muhammad Ali's daughters arrived at his home wearing clothes that were quite revealing. Here is the story as told by one of his daughters:

"When we finally arrived, the chauffeur escorted my younger sister, Laila, and me up to my father's suite. As usual, he was hiding behind the door waiting to scare us. We exchanged as many hugs and kisses as we could possibly give in one day.

My father took a good look at us. Then he sat me down on his lap and said something that I will never forget. He looked me straight in the eyes and said, "Hana, everything that God made valuable in the world is covered and hard to get to.

Where do you find diamonds? Deep down in the ground, covered and protected.

Where do you find pearls?

Deep down at the bottom of the ocean, covered up and protected in a beautiful shell.

Where do you find gold? Way down in the mine, covered over with layers and layers of rock. You've got to work hard to get to them."

He looked at me with serious eyes. "Your body is sacred. You're far more precious than diamonds and pearls, and you should be covered too."

From the book: More Than a Hero: Muhammad Ali's Life Lessons through His Daughter's Eyes

Respect of Your Attitude – There's nothing more disrespectful than a stinky attitude. Unfortunately, it has become the norm and has been accepted for a young woman to have a bad attitude. However, as a Godly young woman, you need to be an exception to the rule. Just because you feel bad doesn't mean you have a right to treat others poorly. There is a time and place for everything and not everybody needs to encounter the wrath of your bad mood. Control your attitude and only put your best foot forward. I have always been told by others that I have a great attitude and I pride myself in treating people with kindness, regardless of my situation, because nobody deserves to be disrespected just because I'm having a mood swing or a bad day. And yes, when I have been caught off guard a time or two (smile), I have apologized to my victims.

Respect of Your Temper – Many young people are incarcerated because their tempers got the best of them. Instead of cooling down to think rationally, they let their temper rage and said and did things, to the point of death, which can't be retracted. These quick lapses in judgment have left a lot of young people dead, paralyzed, and in prison because of acting irrational over a situation that could have been handled through conversation with cooler heads. *"I had a bad temper that was sometimes uncontrollable, only because I failed to control it. I felt that if I was upset I had a right to lash out at my victim however I chose to, be it verbally or physically, and because I was angry I was completely justified in doing so."* However, that's not the right way to handle a situation. The best thing you can do for yourself and the person you are angry with is calm down so you can think things through rationally, to talk rationally about the situation. *Proverbs 29:11 - NIV, "Fools give full vent to their rage, but the wise bring calm in the end."* I know it's easier said than done, but it beats the alternative of doing something you will later regret.

Respect Of Your Spirit – Your spirit is your inner being that displays who you are on the outside. In order to have a good aura *(impression)*, you need to listen to, read, and embrace positive, uplifting, soul quenching spiritual substance. You have to stop feeding your spirit negativity by listening to offensive music with derogatory language, looking at degrading videos, and taking bad advice from friends who don't know any more than you do. *You have to purposely seek out good things and guard your spirit from bad things, places, and even people. Proverbs 4:23-NIV, "Above all else, guard your heart, for everything you do flows from it."* If you feed your spirit on a regular basis with good, sound sustenance (*the Word of God*), you can't help but have a positive, self-respecting aura.

Respect of Your Atmosphere/Family – *Divine Daughter*, you have a great calling in your life as a potential wife and mother. Part of that calling is providing an atmosphere that is pleasing unto God, whether it's in your parent's home or your own home. A young woman sets the atmosphere for her surroundings and is the primary person to make sure things in the home are decent and in order. *There are some things that a woman just does better than a man and making a house a home is one of them (most of the time; there are exceptions to the rule).* More often than not, a woman's value is validated by how well she keeps her home and cares for her children *(not saying it's right, just stating what it is).* *"As a young girl growing up, my mother taught me how to cook, clean, and wash and iron clothes. Not to become Suzy Homemaker, per se, but to build my worth as a woman, so I would know how to take care of myself and manage my family and household when the time arose."* It's not cute not knowing how to care for yourself and eventually your family. There are certain life skills you need to know to elevate your value as a Godly young woman and taking care of your home and family is one of them.

Nowadays, there is a lack of respect and pride for the care of the home environments and children.

As a Godly young woman, you should take pride in keeping your home clean and free of filth. Most often, as the primary homemaker, you need to make it as pleasant as possible, not only for yourself, but for your future husband and children. Not everybody has the gift of decorating, but we can all have the gift of being clean and tidy. In the same token, your children are a reflection of you and your care for them. Keeping them clean and well groomed, well-nourished, and healthy is something you should take pleasure in as a mother, if and when the time comes.

Other Areas of Respect:

- **Physical Respect** - Respect personal boundaries, touch others appropriately, and refrain from violence.

- **Emotional Respect** - Respect other people's feelings and emotions and take responsibility for your own.

- **Verbal Respect** - Be honest; use respectful forms of communication with others, and hear what others are saying to you.

- **Respect of Space** - Respect your own and others' right to privacy, solitude, and peace in their personal space, and negotiate the use of common space. *This is very important in college life.*

- **Respect of Property** - Care for individual, common, and community property.

- **Respect of Differences** - Respect the diversity of people's age, gender, racial origin, sexual orientation, spiritual practices, and physical and mental capabilities.

- **Respect of Rules/Regulations** - Respect the community structure and decision-making process.

Questions/Reflection

1) What is the first rule of respect?

_____

_____

_____

2) How do you respect your elders?

_____

_____

_____

3) What does it mean by respecting your appearance?

_____

_____

_____

4) How do you respect your temper?

_____

_____

_____

5) What are some things to do to respect your spirit?

_____

_____

_____

6) How would you define physical respect?

_____

_____

_____

7) What are some other areas of respect? Explain.

_____

_____

_____

8) Self Reflection: In what ways am I respectful? What areas do I need to work on?

_____

_____

_____

three

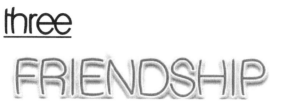

People who lift you up, challenge, encourage, and hold you accountable

Friends; How Many Of Us Have Them?

There are "friends" who destroy each other, but a real friend sticks closer than a brother. *Proverbs 18:24 - NLT*

Dear Divine Daughter,

Everybody cannot be and is not your friend; true friends are hard to find. *You have to pick your friends and not let your friends pick you.* The danger of letting your friends pick you is not knowing who or what you're associating yourself with and the added stress of peer pressure *(social pressure to adopt a type of behavior, dress, or attitude in order to be accepted),* of always trying to live up to their principles and expectations instead of them already being aligned with yours. When you choose your friends, you know what path you are going down because you <u>should choose</u> someone with similar interests and values. When they choose you, they may take you on a journey that's not befitting of your values, who you are or will become.

Short Story: *My freshman year in high school I transferred to a new school and didn't know anybody. I met this young woman in one of my classes and she seemed nice enough and I was just happy to have someone to talk to and hang out with. We would meet up during period changes and have lunch together when we could. She was really friendly and nice.*

After a couple of weeks of these exchanges, I started noticing people looking at me and whispering when I was with her and I found this quite strange. I also started to notice that she really didn't have any other friends and that guys would make these demeaning gestures towards her when walking down the halls. Finally, another young lady from one of my other classes asked me how I knew her and I said we just met in one of my classes. She went on to tell me that the young woman was bad news and there were rumors going around the school that she had been sexually active with several football players and even had a baby. By her befriending me and me not knowing anything about her, I got associated with her reputation. The reason they were looking at me was to see if I was like her (birds of a feather flock together). The rumors I heard were disturbing because I really liked her as a person. But, after getting to know her better, she wasn't a person I could keep as a friend because we were going in different directions with a completely different mindset.

When choosing a friend, you have to determine what qualities you want in a friend. They say birds of a feather flock together; make sure you're associating with the right flock. There have been many people sent to prison because of their association with so-called friends. Some might say, just because she's my friend doesn't mean I have to do what she does. The problem with that statement is why is she your friend if you are going in two different directions? The young woman, in my situation, was a nice person, but we couldn't be friends. Not because of her past *(we all make mistakes),* but because of where she was going in her future, which was further down the same destructive path. Understand, you have friends and you have associates. A friendship is a tried and tested relationship. You have to know that person is true to you, has your back, and is similar to who you are morally. An associate is just someone you associate with because of a class or job, church or community service activities you might have together, or it could be a family member, but that is the extent of your relationship *(take note: all family members are not your friends – you can't choose who you are related to, but you can choose who your friends are).*

In life, you will have good and bad experiences finding true friendship. Growing up, I had more than a few bad experiences with so-called friends. It's not easy to know who your true friends are until you're put in a situation with your back against the wall and you see who's there fighting with you and who's standing against you. Many times we are too trusting of a person before we really get to know their true character, *who they are when no one is looking*. I have learned that it's better to watch what a person does than only to pay attention to what they say. In other words, their words need to line up with their actions. If you tell me you're one way, but I see you treating your other friends a different way, I know you're not a person of integrity or honesty. If you talk about your other friends to me, then I know for sure you're talking about me to them; that's part of your character, *what you do when you think no one else is watching*. When choosing friendships, your potential friends have to show/prove their sincerity or get the boot. The way you test whether a person is truly friend material is by testing and watching how they handle certain situations.

To assess whether they're trustworthy, you can entrust them with a small secret *(nothing crucially important)* to see whether or not it gets back to you. If you wait a couple of weeks and none of your mutual friends or associates mentions anything to you, you know you can be a little more trusting. Test them again, this time with something a little more important *(nothing that can hurt you if it gets out)* to see if they kept it to themselves. If after a couple of weeks nothing comes back, you know that person <u>has the potential</u> to be trustworthy. However, building a trustworthy friendship is a gradual process and happens over time. You have to be conscious of the exchanges you have with this potential friend to determine if they are true friend material. You need to look for the following:

Compatibility: You want a friend who shares similar goals, interests, and hobbies. You need friends who are going in the same Godly direction as you, so you can support and keep each other on track. Opposite of this: Someone who tries to compete with you in a mean-spirited way or try to make you jealous, or try to get you to do something wrong.

Communicative: You want a friend with whom you can talk to about anything and that actually listens and tries to understand your viewpoint, even if they disagree. You also want someone with whom you can talk through negative feelings of anger to work out an unpleasant situation.

Considerate: You want a friend who really cares about you and others around them. Never have a friend who gives nothing of themselves to the relationship. Being a friend is giving and taking in balance, not one always giving and the other always taking.

Enjoyable: You want a friend whom you enjoy being around, to laugh, have fun, and just be silly.

Integrity: You want a friend who is honest and does what they say they're going to do.

Loyal: You want someone whom you respect and who respects you, who is there for you and has your back. Not everyone who says they're your friend will be there for you.

Optimistic: You want a friend that has a positive outlook on life and isn't doom and gloom all the time. You want someone who's happy when you succeed or happy about something just because you're happy about it.

Progressing: You want a friend who can accompany you on the journey to personal growth. You want someone who is always working on being a better person and inspires and motivates you to be better. Some friends are only for a season of time in your life, because when you're elevating and trying to do something better or different, they might not be able to catch that train with you because your mindsets have become different. As you get older and develop more friendships, you need to have a friend who is younger so you can help and encourage, one who is around the same age so you can relate and encourage each other, and one who is older who can help and encourage you.

Trustworthy: You want a friend you can trust with your secrets and feelings, who won't gossip about you. You also want a friend who is sensitive to your feelings, but will always be truthful with you and have your best interest in mind.

It is very difficult to cultivate friendships with all the cattiness *(meanness)* and jealousy between young women. When you truly find someone who cares about you and your well-being, you need to cherish that relationship and reciprocate the same qualities you want in a friendship because good friends are hard to find.

Questions/Reflection

1) How do you choose a friend?

_____
_____
_____

2) What are some characteristics of a friend?

_____
_____
_____

3) What type of friends should you have?

_____
_____
_____

4) Why is it not good for someone to choose you as a friend, without you choosing them?

_____
_____
_____

5) What's the difference between a friend and associate?

_____
_____
_____

6) What are the characteristics of a bad friend?

_____
_____
_____

7) Self-Reflection: What kind of friend are you? In what areas can you be a better friend?

_____
_____
_____

four

HYGIENE

Cleanliness Is Next To Godliness

"I beseech you therefore, brethren, by the mercies of God, that ye present your bodies a living sacrifice, holy, acceptable unto God, which is your reasonable service."
Romans 12:1- KJV

Dear Divine Daughter,

Your body is a temple to be treasured, and as a young woman, there are many things you need to know to properly care for your body, so listen up:

General Hygiene

First of all, you need to wash your hands often throughout the day. The following are times when it's really important to wash or sanitize your hands *(carry hand sanitizer; you will not always be near soap and water)*:

- Before/During/After Food Preparation

- Before/After eating

- After blowing your nose, coughing, or sneezing

- After using the bathroom or changing sanitary pad/tampon

- After changing diapers

- After touching animals

- After touching unclean objects *(trash, grocery carts, door handles, keyboards, cell phones, etc.)*

- Before/After touching or cleaning open sores

Being aware of what you're touching, and sanitizing where appropriate, will greatly reduce the transference of colds and bacteria that cause illness.

Body Cleansing

As a female, you have a lot of crevices that perspire and cause body odor, so you need to bathe/shower on a daily basis. It is important that you wash your entire body daily with a shower gel or bar of soap using a bath sponge or wash cloth making sure to wash all over, especially under the arms, under the breasts, and the genital area *(use a vaginal wash for this area – some soaps can be too harsh)*.

> When wiping the genital area, always wipe from front to back to reduce bacterial infections. You can reach around back and start at the front of the genitals and wipe back toward the anus.

If you play sports or have a highly active lifestyle, wash as often as needed. After showering/bathing, consider moisturizing your skin with a good absorbent lotion or oil so your skin stays soft and smooth, to avoid dry, cracked, and eventually, wrinkled skin.

It's also a good idea to wear an antiperspirant deodorant and to keep your underarms shaved to reduce holding perspiration, odor, and the appearance of caked deodorant. Although shaving under your arms, as well as shaving your legs are optional and a personal preference, *in my personal opinion,* you look more polished if these areas are shaved.

Menstrual Cycle

During your puberty years *(11-16, give or take a few years)* you will experience a change in your body hormones based on the beginning of menstruation *(the monthly process of discharging blood and other matter from the womb).* This defines the moment in your life when you have transitioned from little girl to young woman because now you have the ability to conceive children. It may come as a shock to see blood coming from your most private part, but this is just the start of a very long, uncomfortable, monthly relationship with your companion called the period, TOM (Time Of Month), menstrual cycle, or your girlfriend *(which is what I call mine).* During this time, you may experience PMS (Premenstrual Syndrome) which includes, but is not limited to, the following:

- Moodiness
- Difficulty sleeping

- Bloating (Fluid retention)
- Nervousness
- Cravings (for me, its chocolate; got to have it)

You may have no pain at all but some may experience the following:

- Leg aches
- Back pain
- Stomach cramps
- Queasiness
- Diarrhea
- Tiredness

The pain might be so severe that some may need to take pain relievers during this time and use a heating pad to ease cramping. The menstruation period usually last from three to seven days *(everyone is different)* and flows vary from really heavy in the beginning to light or spotty at the end. It is very important that you pay close attention to your hygiene because the discharge often has a very unpleasant odor and requires you to change your tampon/pad every four to eight hours, maybe even sooner depending on your flow and activity level.

When choosing a feminine product to absorb the moisture, you might have to try out a few to see what's comfortable for you. There are many sanitary products on the market, but the most unique difference is whether you use a **tampon** *(a tubular plug of soft material <u>inserted in the vagina</u> during menstruation to absorb moisture)* or a **sanitary pad/napkin** *(a strip of absorbent material that sticks to your underwear, that is used <u>externally</u> to absorb the moisture)*.

Both methods are effective in absorbing the moisture, but with the tampon you might need to combine usage with a panty liner *(a really thin version of a sanitary pad)* for minor leakage during the heavy flow times. You can also use panty liners when you're at the end of your menstrual period and just spotting instead of using a tampon or full size pad. You will also need to make sure you keep your vaginal area clean and fresh in between changing your tampon/pad with vaginal wipes. There are many brands on the market to keep you smelling fresh and clean during this time as well as on an everyday basis. Also, be sure to keep extra sanitary products with you at all times; you never know when you may need it. It is always good to be prepared.

Please Note: Because the tampon is inserted inside the vagina, the fibers it's made from can sometimes cause Toxic Shock Syndrome (TSS), which is a rare, but serious infection that occurs when toxins made by certain strains of Staphylococcus aureus bacteria (Staph) get into the bloodstream. The initial symptoms are similar to the flu, and can include high fever, nausea, vomiting, diarrhea, dizziness, fainting, and disorientation. It is important to change your tampon every four to eight hours. Do not use them overnight.

Yeast Infections

A yeast infection is a common, sometimes reoccurring, infection that comes when too many yeast cells are growing in the vagina, which is caused by a type of yeast called Candida. The overgrowth of yeast could be due to changing hormones, medications, a medical condition, etc. The symptoms of a yeast infection are itching or soreness in the vagina that sometimes causes pain or burning when you urinate. Some may even have a thick, clumpy, white discharge that has no odor and looks a little like cottage cheese. These symptoms are more likely to occur during the week before your menstrual period.

If you have a yeast infection, it can be treated by using an over the counter medication such as an antifungal cream or suppository that you insert into your vagina.

If this is your first time experiencing these symptoms, please see your family physician to get an accurate diagnosis.

To prevent future yeast infections, take heed to the following:

- Keep your vaginal area clean. Use a mild, unscented vaginal wash and rinse well.

- After using the toilet, wipe from front to back to avoid spreading yeast or bacteria from your anus to the vagina or urinary tract.

- Wear underwear that helps keep your genital area dry and doesn't hold in warmth and moisture. A good choice is cotton underwear.

- Avoid tight-fitting clothing, such as pantyhose and tight-fitting jeans. These may increase body heat and moisture in your genital area.

- Change out of wet swimsuits right away. Wearing a wet swimsuit for many hours may keep your genital area warm and moist.

- Change pads or tampons often.

- Don't douche or use deodorant tampons or feminine sprays, powders, or perfumes. These items can change the normal balance of organisms in your vagina.

Hair

Hair is one thing, as you mature, you will begin to take pride in showing off. However, it is very easy to get caught up in the latest hairstyles without taking proper care of your hair, by using harsh chemicals, dyes, weaves *(extensions)*, wigs, bonding glue, and curling irons. Since hair differs by texture, length, and thickness, there's not a one-size-fits-all method. For basic hygiene, you or a stylist need to shampoo *(lather the shampoo in your hair, gently scrub scalp with fingertips, rinse with warm water, then repeat the process)*, condition *(choose a conditioner based on your hair type to maximize its potential),* and moisturizer as your hair type dictates *(if it's oily – wash more often and use less/no moisturizer; if it's dry – wash less often and moisturize when needed)*. You need to be very careful not to damage your hair by using a flat/curling iron at high temperatures daily. You will also need to make sure your hair ends are cut often *(at least every six to eight weeks or as needed)* to keep hair healthy, to prevent split ends and breakage. Take the time to care for your hair; it is one of the characteristics that express a young woman's features.

Face

You need to take time to care for your face. Since young women are wearing make-up at an earlier age, and lot more of it, not taking care of your face can make you look a lot older and cause your skin to blemish. It's important to clean your face daily with a cleanser for your skin type, whether dry, oily, or combination and moisturize accordingly with an SPF 15 or higher moisturizer to protect your skin from the sun. Your skin looks good now, but keep on living and you'll need some supplements to keep it looking good for the long haul.

Oral Hygiene

Your mouth harbors a lot of bacteria due to the different foods, candy, drinks, and spices consumed daily. You need to brush after each meal *(or at the very least, twice a day, morning and night, with an anti-cavity toothpaste)* and floss between teeth to keep bacteria from developing cavities, an odor, or worse, an infection in your mouth. You will need to change your toothbrush often *(about every three months)*, especially when or before signs of wear are evident, i.e. bristles fanning out or flattening. A pleasant smile that shows your pearly whites is a big asset to have as a young woman. No one wants to see or smell a yucky mouth.

Nails

Another area to take extra care in maintaining is your nails. Make sure your fingernails and toenails are clean and free of dirt *(if your nails are dirty, it makes your whole body look dirty/unclean)*. If you wear polish, make sure it's not cracked, chipped, or peeling; this, too, looks very unattractive and messy. If you have trouble maintaining your feet or hands on your own, a twice monthly mani/pedi would help assist in the upkeep of appearance *(it'll be a good treat to work toward)*.

Questions/Reflection

1) How often should you bathe?

_____

_____

_____

2) How should you wipe the genital area after using the restroom?

_____

_____

_____

3) What are three occasions to wash your hands?

_____

_____

_____

4) How many times daily should you brush your teeth?

_____

_____

_____

5) What's the difference between a tampon and sanitary pad?

_____

_____

_____

6) How often should your hair be trimmed?

_____

_____

_____

7) Self-Reflection: What areas need improvement? How do I plan to improve them?

_____

_____

_____

five

DATING &
RELATIONSHIPS

Don't Give Him the Benefits of a Husband When He's Not Asking You to Be His Wife

Do not be conformed to this world, but be transformed by the renewal of your mind, that by testing you may discern what is the will of God, what is good and acceptable and perfect. *Romans 12:2-ESV*

Dear Divine Daughter,

Dating and Relationships are a very big deal to young women. Many are confused about when a young man is truly in to them. Some force themselves on young men. Others feel they can't live without a young man. In my day we called them boy-crazy. Then you have some who feel that if they give themselves over to young men to be used or abused, they will be loved. *This often happens when you don't know your worth*.

When you date someone it is an act of getting to know the other person's moral values and character, their personality, their hopes and dreams, and their life plans, just to see if your mindsets and goals are compatible. Nowadays, young people consider dating as a time to hookup and have sexual relations without taking the time to explore whether or not that person is right for them, to develop a friendship before trying to cultivate a relationship. It's sad that young people are hooking up and having babies with people they really don't even know. If you knew your self-worth, you would know that no one is meant to know you intimately except your husband. I know you're saying that's old fashioned and people don't stay virgins until their married anymore. It's the 21st century and that's the way it's done. But I ask you, **_What does God say?_** I find that we have generations of mistakes because we did it our way or the world's way, but not God's way. You have a chance to start out the right way; to not go through a lot of heartache and pain or to bring children into the world without stable homes. You have a chance to do it God's way and reap the blessings that come with doing it His way. I know many of you have a heart's desire to do it God's way and will date without sleeping around, will wait for the man that chooses you to be his wife, will be a virgin on the night you get married, and will bear children by your husband only. But I also know there are some who will not wait. We get swept away by the romance and choose not to do it God's way for one reason or another. Here are some things to consider before you make that decision, so listen up:

"Don't be Rented When Looking for a Buyer"

When an apartment is rented, you pay to stay. You are only responsible for partial upkeep (*only doing what's required*) while there for six or twelve months. You don't have to cut the yard, fix things when they break, or worry about the property value. There is no long term commitment to renting because the place is being used constantly by other people. Usually, when someone rents a place, they don't treat it like it's their own, so therefore, they don't really care about the upkeep because they can leave once their lease is up or when they want to. This is what happens when you're in a **Renter's Relationship -** *He only wants to be with you to get what he wants without making a long term commitment to care for your overall needs. He doesn't bring anything to the relationship but his appetite and uses you for his benefit, while only doing what's required to keep you interested in fulfilling his needs. When he's done, bored and tired of you, he moves on to find someone else to rent.*

On the other hand, when you buy a home you enter into a long term contract and commit yourself to total upkeep of the property. If something is broken, you fix it. You can't just leave at any time, because you made a commitment to maintain the property; you are totally responsible for it. This is what happens when you're in a **Buyer's Relationship** *–He's not with you for what he can get; he's there to care about your total well-being and wants to care for all of your wants and needs. He brings more to the relationship than just his appetite and does what's required to keep you satisfied. After he has cultivated a friendship and is ready to move to the next level, he puts a ring on your finger and asks for your hand in marriage, not to sleep with you.*

You need to know the difference because if you're constantly in a renter's relationship, you'll never get a buyer. Make sure you get a God-sent buyer and not a Satan-filled renter. Many young women get used because they treat their significant other like a buyer when he's only looking to rent. *In other words,* **"don't give him the benefits of a husband when he's not asking you to be his wife."**

It might be the world's norm to have friends with benefits, or to have the occasional booty call, but really and truly, what benefits are you receiving by sharing your body with multiple people who care so little about you they can only commit to you as a friend with the benefit of having sex, or less - just a sex partner? This type of behavior, more often than not, produces baby mamas – mamas without a husband. There are so many baby mamas that it's become the norm to have a baby without being married, to have sexually transmitted diseases (STDs), and to have impure spirits due to all the people who have had sex with you. ***When you're being rented, you are constantly being used. A worn out place rarely gets a buyer.***

The growing trend of friends with benefits and booty calls has caused breaks in the family unit. This behavior produces a result of fatherless children and denies them the privilege to grow up in the safe and healthy environment that is needed to become a functional, wholesome adult. God did not design the family unit to consist of a mother and her children. He designed it to have a mother and a father to guide and lead their children in the way they should go. *Proverbs 22:6 – KJV, Train up a child in the way he should go: and when he is old, he will not depart from it.* You should never put yourself in such an unsecure situation. I know we don't always do what's right and we sometimes make mistakes.

When you know better, you need to do better.

Divine Daughter, I tell you this not to be scornful or old-fashion, but to let you know that the street named "Friends w/Benefits" at the intersection of "Booty Call" is not one you want to go down and it will ultimately only lead to problems. If you find yourself in a situation of being a baby mama, at least make the best of the situation by doing these things:

Make Your Child/Children A Priority – Having a child/children without being married is going to leave you and the child/children in a vulnerable situation. You will be the main provider emotionally and most times financially- if you're lucky you might receive a little child support. This is going to be very stressful. The child with only one parent and provider sometimes has a void in their lives causing self-hate. A child may feel as if it's their fault when one parent is not in their life. They feel devalued. A child may feel worthless when they don't have the love and support of both parents because all their needs are not being met – one parent can't do it alone; it takes two, along with a village. They often feel unlovable when there's only one parent providing support emotionally and financially; one area goes lacking and often it's the emotional aspect. You have no choice but to provide for their needs, food, shelter, and clothing, but many single parents are too drained from providing financially to give emotional care. *You have to make your children a priority; they did not ask to be here or to be put in this situation.* Whatever free time you have needs to be spent educating them and encouraging them to do their best, teaching them morals and values, disciplining them in love according to their age (*no abuse;*

know the difference and don't let anyone else be abusive to them, i.e. new boyfriends), and loving them unconditionally. Don't let the TV or gaming devices be their babysitter or their teacher. Build a cocoon of loving, trusting caregivers to help you guide your child/children in the right direction, be it grandparents, aunts or uncles.

Don't Bring Everyone You Meet Around Your Child/Children – Not everyone is qualified to meet or greet your child/children. The only time your child/children should meet someone you're dating is when you are seriously thinking about marriage *(make sure he's a buyer and not a renter)*. Then, and only then, should you introduce him to your child/children so they can start developing a relationship. Be aware of how your child/children react to this person because children are generally good judges of character. They can often sense whether a person is good or has a hidden agenda. Kids can genuinely tell when someone is sincere, so be watchful and pay close attention to their interactions with this person because the worst thing you can do is put your child/children in harm's way, whether verbal, physical, or sexual. The world is a crazy place. If possible, run a background check. You can never be too careful, especially when it comes to your children.

Don't Invest Your Time Looking For A Mate – Mothers, both young and old, go out looking for a man when they should allow a **man** to look for them. Men like to be the aggressors in the relationship, meaning they like to pursue you, not have you pursue them. When you pursue a man you look desperate and looking desperate can lead to you being taken advantage of by the wrong man. If you invest your time in advancing yourself and your child/children, when that special someone does come into your life, you have something to offer besides baggage.

Don't Have Sex Without Being Married – Ok, this statement alone should be enough said considering the situation you're already in *(baby mama status)*. If you continue with this behavior of having sex with a renter instead of your buyer *(husband)*, you will only produce more children without being married, which makes it difficult for your husband *(buyer)* to find you. It's no man's desire to deal with a woman with multiple baby daddies. *Remember, a worn out place rarely gets a buyer.* When you're dating someone, sex should not be mandatory or a priority. If the person you're dating is serious about a relationship with you, he will respect your **no sex rule** and use the time you share together to get to know you on a personal, not sexual, level. If he doesn't, he wasn't serious about you and was just looking for sex. True love is given without expecting anything in return. If he doesn't understand this, keep it moving... and don't look back!

Stop Settling For A Nickel When You're A Dime (Lowering Your Standards); If You're A Nickel, Become A Dime (Elevate Your Status) – *Don't hook up with the first boy/man that shows interest in you just to say you have someone.* You need to know your worth and stop settling for the first good-looking, smooth talking boy/man with the swag you like that steps to you. You have to be particular about who you choose as a mate and pray for God's guidance in selecting the right one. Having a child/children doesn't make you worthless. You want someone who is <u>truly</u> seeking/nurturing a personal relationship with God, has similar morals and values, treats you well, is a man of his word – does what he says he will do, loves you inside and out, confident, independent, has plans/goals for a good future-progressing, appreciative, loyal, honest, cherishes your child/children, and can be supportive emotionally, financially, and physically.

You also have to bring more to the relationship than just your appetite. You have to have something of worth to offer as well. You have to be on a path of self-progression, whether pursuing a college education or career path. You have to have something going on besides just going out. You need to <u>truly</u> be seeking/nurturing a personal relationship with God, be emotionally stable (no bad attitude or flipping out over nothing), patient, loyal, self-sufficient, responsible, supportive, a good homemaker and in a position of already taking care of your business and your child/children so when your mate does come along he is an asset to your situation, and you're not a decline to his.

Now, if you're <u>not</u> a baby mama, but you're participating in "friends with benefits" or "booty call" behavior, you need to evaluate these behaviors before continuing or starting this destructive conduct. First, know this: Everything the world shows you might look good to you, but it's not always good for you, so listen up:

Don't Share Your Body With Everybody And Leave Your Future Husband The Leftovers – *Divine Daughter*, you give the best part of your body away when you don't wait for your husband. Since the beginning of time, sex was meant to be between a husband and wife. Because the world has detoured from that, we have many fatherless children, broken homes, teenage pregnancies, and STDs (Sexually Transmitted Diseases). Every time you have sex with someone, you're allowing their spirit to connect and occupy your spiritual being for a lifetime. How many spirits will you, or have you, mixed with yours for a lifetime? Is it or was it worth it?

Stop Having Sex Like You Are Married, But Not Willing Or Able To Handle The Responsibilities That A Married Couple Has To Handle When And If A Child Is Conceived The fact of the matter is this lack of responsibility causes children to suffer because many times they are stuck in a situation that is unstable due to having young parents with no job, no education, or means of support. Families have to step in and help raise the child/children and some families are not prepared or inclined to raise another generation of children after raising their own. This situation may cause resentment in the family unit which sometimes leads to a lack of nurturing and love for the child/children. This produces another lost generation who will not be taught the values of life. You had better think about it. *Is it worth it?*

Don't Have Unprotected Sex (Oral, Anal, Or Vaginal) With Anyone – Having sex with multiple partners unprotected will only increase your chances of contracting or transmitting a STD and it might be one you have to live with for the rest of your life.

Your Body Was Created To Give Life, To Be Nurturing And For Love *(specifically for your husband)*, not to be passed from person to person for sexual pleasure.

Your Body Is Not For A Young Man To Have His Way With You, only to lust after you *(because it has nothing to do with love)* and leave you for his next victim.

Just Because You Have Sex With Him Doesn't Mean He'll Love You Or Want You, You need to respect yourself and your body by waiting for your husband who will love you the right way so you feel secure and truly loved. Don't give away your body so easily just because the first good-looking boy you see says he loves you. If he loves you, let him show you with his actions in front of his family and friends at the altar – not between the sheets. Anybody can say "I love you"; it's his deeds that prove it (show and prove or get the boot). Also, just because he professes his love for you, it doesn't mean you have to reward him with your body.

It Is Important For You To Know It's Okay To Wait Until You Are Married To Have Sex
It's not always easy to wait because of outside influence and your raging hormones, but if you make up your mind that you want the best for your life and you want to do it God's way, you will do your best to wait. *When you put yourself in adult situations, you have to be prepared for adult responsibilities.* You might think marriage no longer has value because of the high divorce rate, but many of those marriages lacked the foundation *(rooting their marriage on and in the Word of God)* it takes to have a stable relationship because their priorities were not right. You have to really understand and mean the vows you take for a marriage to last. You cannot enter with phony expectations and think things will fall into place by themselves; it takes

hard work daily to make it work. If you work hard, you will be truly blessed.

Abusive Relationships

Divine Daughter, more and more young people are entering abusive relationships. About one in three young adults know someone who has been hit by a boyfriend or girlfriend, girls can be abusive too. As I said so many times before, you are precious in the eyes of God and no one has the right to hurt you. You need to recognize that abuse is the result of one person trying to have control over another and it can be physical, psychological *(emotional),* or both. No one has the right to put their hands on you or to harm you in any manner. Here are some things to look for regarding physical and emotional abuse:

Physical Abuse:

- Scratching, slapping, punching, biting, strangling, or kicking

- Throwing something at you, such as a phone, book, shoe, etc.

- Pulling your hair

- Pushing or pulling you

- Grabbing your clothing

- Using a gun, knife, box cutter, bat, mace, or other weapon

- Forcing you to have sex or perform a sexual act

- Grabbing your face to make you look at them

- Grabbing you to prevent you from leaving or to force you to go somewhere

Psychological (Emotional) Abuse:

- Putting you down

- Making you feel bad about yourself

- Name calling

- Playing mind games; making you think you're being irrational

- Humiliating you

- Making you feel guilty about something they did to you

If you are in a relationship and notice these signs, you need to:

- Realize this behavior is wrong

- Not accept or make excuses for this abusive behavior

- Talk to an adult, friend, or family member that you trust to get help

- Create a safety plan to get out of the situation

- Consider getting a restraining order, if needed

Remember there is no justification for abuse; it's not your fault.

Questions/Reflection

1) Why is it important to wait until you're married to have sex with someone?

_____

_____

_____

2) What's the difference between a renter and buyer?

_____

_____

_____

3) What are some things you need to do if you're in baby mama status?

_____

_____

_____

4) When is it appropriate for someone to meet your child/children?

_____

_____

_____

5) What do you do while you're waiting for your God-sent mate?

_____

_____

_____

6) What is the best way for someone to show you they love you?

_____

_____

_____

7) What are some signs that someone is abusive?

_____

_____

_____

8) Self-Reflection: Do you want to be in baby mama status? What steps will you take to do what is pleasing to God?

_____

_____

_____

six

Let's Talk About Sex...

Flee from sexual immorality. All other sins a person commits are outside the body, but whoever sins sexually, sins against their own body. [19] Do you not know that your bodies are temples of the Holy Spirit, who is in you, whom you have received from God? You are not your own; [20] you were bought at a price. Therefore honor God with your bodies. - *1 Corinthians 6:18 - 20-NIV*

DISCLAIMER: This is a very sensitive topic and, if at all possible, should be discussed with a parent or guardian in more detail. I will give a general overview of what sex involves, being straightforward with the information, to lessen confusion and reveal knowledge for better decision making.

Dear Divine Daughter,

Please know that sex is an intimate act that God ordained as good to be shared between a <u>husband</u> and <u>wife</u> for the reproduction of children and lovemaking. He did not ordain it as a random act between two strangers or friends for pleasure.

Basics of Sex

Sex is physical contact with the male genitalia (penis) using hands, mouth, anus, or female genitalia (vagina).

As you get older and start maturing into a young woman, your body goes in to a stage called puberty. During puberty there are several changes that take place in your body, like: hair growth under the arms and genital region, breast growth, sweat production, oily skin or acne, along with sexual feelings and thoughts. It is also the start of menstruation, as we discussed in the hygiene section. I mentioned that when you start your menstrual cycle you become a young woman because now you can get pregnant.

Let's discuss how pregnancy happens. When a man and woman have sex, the man inserts his erect penis inside the woman's vagina; semen, a milky fluid containing sperm, comes out of the man's penis through ejaculation, which enters the woman's vagina. Once in the vagina, the sperm travels through the cervix *(opening to the womb)* into the uterus *(womb)* and then into the fallopian tubes *(egg canals)* where it connects with the woman's egg. This is called fertilization. Once fertilization takes place, and the fertilized egg travels down the fallopian tube and attaches itself to the wall of the uterus, you are pregnant. It only takes <u>one</u> sexual encounter for pregnancy to happen. This is the physical side of procreation and sex. Sex also has a spiritual and emotional side.

Before there were weddings and marriage licenses, men and women were only considered to be legally married once they consummated *(to come together sexually to combine two spirits into one)* their marriage. *Genesis 2:24-KJV, "Therefore shall a man leave his father and his mother, and shall cleave unto his wife and they shall be one flesh."* If they didn't consummate their marriage, their marriage could be annulled *(canceled)* as if it never happened. When a man and woman come together sexually, they become a part of each other's spirit. This is the most intimate exchange two people can have and at that point of connection their spirits interconnect and they can become a part of one another for a lifetime. This means you are connected to that person because that sexual encounter connected your emotions and spirits together, creating a soul tie. A soul tie is a linkage in the spiritual realm between two people. It links their spirits together, which can bring forth both negative (tainted/abused) and positive (marriage/soul mate) results. This also means, if you have had past sexual relationships, you have soul ties with those spirits and everyone they have had sexual encounters with as well, and vice versa; they are connected with everyone you have had sex with in the past. This behavior can create a lot of baggage in the form of having all those spirits (soul ties) connected to yours. These soul ties usually show up in the form of a comparison of sexual encounters you have had with past partners to your present relationship, fantasizing about sexual experiences with past sexual partners, romanticizing past relationships or being traumatized by bad abusive sexual experiences with someone.

The emotional aspect of this exchange is overwhelming because young women see things differently than young men do. A sexual exchange for a young woman brings about a connection of intimate feelings of love and closeness, but for a young man, it is what it is. It's just a sexual encounter; nothing more, nothing less. This opposite reaction of emotions often leaves the female yearning for love and the male yearning for sex, which is why so often, females have sex to *get the feeling of receiving love* and males show affection *(not love)* to get sex.

Sex is such a big deal in society today. Every time you turn on the television you see some kind of sexual display in commercials, nightly sitcoms, music videos, movies, etc. It's as if you can't get away from it. Many young women are being influenced by so-called friends and boyfriends to have sex or worse, to have babies *(pregnancy pacts)* while unmarried with no job or place to raise a family.

Being a *Divine Daughter* you are called to a higher standard of living that is much different than the world would have you live. The world says if it feels good, just do it. But God says everything has to be done decent and in order. *1 Corinthians 14:40 - KJV, "Let all things be done decently and in order".* Many of you might have experienced, talked about, or have been curious about sex and wanted to know what all the hype was about. Let me tell you about sex, God's way vs. the world's way. First, God's way is to make love to your husband and the world's way is to have sex with whomever. The world's way says "What's love got to do with it." God's way says love has **everything** to do with it.

Sex the World's Way	Love God's Way
If You Really Like/Love the Person, Do It	**No Pre-Marital Sex**
It's Okay to be Just a Baby Mama	**No Children Before Marriage**
You're Free to Have a Sexual Relationship with Whomever You Want	**Each Man Shall Have His Own Wife And Wife Her Own Husband**

Sex the World's Way

If You Really Like/Love the Person, Do It

The world says if you really like/love a person and they really like/love you, it's okay to have sex. You can use the birth control method of your choice *(morning after/birth control pills, inserts, rhythm method, or abortions)* to protect yourself from having babies and use condoms to prevent STDs, even if those do somehow fail to work occasionally. The problem is we all have a tendency to really like/love someone at some time or another. Many young women have shared their bodies with young men based on "really like/love" only to find out that "really like/love" turned in to "wham, bam, thank you, ma'am," meaning after the guy got what he wanted from you, the use of your body, he moved on to the next person he "really liked/loved".

> **BE NOT DECEIVED. THIS IS NOT LIKE OR LOVE; IT'S LUST**
> (a strong physical desire to have sex with someone)

They might like you as a person and love you as a friend, but the only time you know it's true love is when they put a ring on your finger. Other than that, it's LUST! When it's true love, it's given without expecting anything in return. Please, be responsible with your body, respect its value, and not allow someone to rob you of your most precious gift to your husband, all in the name of ***lust disguised as love***.

Love God's Way

No Pre-Marital Sex

God says your body is only to be shared with your husband after you get married and in that order. God wants you to connect yourself with only the man who has vowed to love, honor, and cherish you in front of Him and your family, not some random guy who couldn't care less about you after you have sex with him. God ordained it this way so you would share your spirit with only your husband, eliminating any baggage of past failed relationships, Sexually Transmitted Diseases (STDs), or babies out of wedlock.

> Many marriages fail for one reason or another, but fail most times because we choose our mate instead of allowing God to choose. The result may be a bad marriage with someone who is abusive, ungodly, or lacks the biblically moral principles to be a husband and father.

Sex the World's Way

It's Okay to be Just a Baby Mama

The world says it's okay to have sex and a baby with someone if you like/love them or barely even know them *(a one night stand, booty call, or hook-up)*, even if they have no intention of ever marrying you. You can have the baby and keep it moving on to the next person you like/love and have a baby for them, too. It doesn't matter if you have three children by three different fathers. You can make the fathers pay child support *(most often they can't or don't even support themselves, much less have a job to support their child/children)* and get on welfare to meet the rest of your needs. It's your prerogative and body; you can do whatever you want, even if your kids don't have a secure, stable environment of financial and emotional support.

Love God's Way

No Children Before Marriage

God says get married first and then have children, in that order. God wants you to have the protection and financial security of a husband in order to raise and provide for a family. This is the order in which God ordained the family unit. He wants the family to consist of a husband/father and a wife/mother for children to have structure and security. The husband/father is the provider, protector, and spiritual guide. The mother is the helpmate helping the father to meet those needs, homemaker, and comforter of the home. When it's done any other way, in most cases, it creates chaos, such as fatherless children, poverty, and disobedient children.

Sex the World's Way

You're Free to Have a Sexual Relationship with Whomever You Want

The world says if they make you feel good in an intimate way, whether male or female, married or single, then it's okay to have a sexual relationship with them. You should always base your actions by how you feel especially if you have a strong feeling about it, because it must be right.

Love God's Way

Each Man Shall Have His Own Wife and Wife Her Own Husband

But since sexual immorality is occurring, each man should have sexual relations with his own wife and each woman with her own husband. 1 Corinthians 7:2 - NIV

God says when you do something it should be done decent and in order. Each man shall have his own wife and each woman shall have her own husband, not each man or woman shall have whomever they desire. God created Adam and Eve, a male and a female, to be joined together in a family union. He didn't ordain homosexuality, fornication, adultery, threesomes, or open marriages. Just because you have strong feelings about somebody doesn't make it right for you to have sex with them.

Sexually Transmitted Diseases (STDs)

Being sexually active with multiple partners leads to disease and infections of the body. Some can be cured with antibiotics; some cannot be cured and you will live with them for the rest of your life. This is why it's always good to do things God's way instead of the world's way; it will cause you a lot less trouble in the end. Below are some common STDs to be aware of:

Disease: **Chlamydia** is a common, sexually transmitted disease (STD) caused by a bacterium. Chlamydia can infect both men and women and can cause serious permanent damage to a woman's reproductive organs. If left untreated it can cause infertility *(will be unable to conceive children)*.

Symptoms: Chlamydia is known as a 'silent' infection because most infected people have no symptoms and they may not appear until several weeks after exposure. Chlamydia can damage a woman's reproductive organs. Some infected women have an abnormal vaginal discharge or a burning sensation when urinating. Untreated infections can spread causing pelvic inflammatory disease (PID).

PID can be silent, or can cause symptoms such as abdominal and pelvic pain.

Cure: Chlamydia can be easily treated and cured with antibiotics.

Disease: Genital Herpes is highly contagious and is caused by a type of the herpes simplex virus (HSV). HSV enters your body through mucous membranes or small breaks in your skin.

Symptoms: The initial symptoms of genital herpes are usually pain or itching around the genital area, buttocks, or inner thighs beginning within a few weeks after exposure to an infected sexual partner. After several days, small, red bumps may appear. They then rupture, becoming ulcers that ooze or bleed. Eventually, scabs form and the ulcers heal.

Cure: There is no treatment that can cure herpes. Antiviral medications can, however, prevent or shorten outbreaks during the period of time the person takes the medication. Daily use of antiviral medication can also reduce the likelihood of transmission to partners.

Disease: <u>Genital Warts</u> may be as small as one millimeter in diameter or may multiply into large clusters. Genital warts can grow on the vulva, the walls of the vagina, the area between the external genitals and the anus, and the cervix. Genital warts can also develop in the mouth or throat of a person who has had oral sex with an infected person.

Symptoms: The signs and symptoms of genital warts include:

- Small, flesh-colored or gray swellings in your genital area

- Several warts close together that take on a cauliflower shape

- Itching or discomfort in your genital area

- Bleeding with intercourse

Cure: There is no treatment for the virus itself, but there are treatments for the problems that it can cause. Visible genital warts may remain the same, grow more numerous, or go away on their own. They can be removed by the patient with medications. They can also be treated by a health care provider.

Disease: Gonorrhea is a sexually transmitted disease caused by a bacterium. Gonorrhea can grow easily in the warm, moist areas of the reproductive tract, including the cervix, uterus, and fallopian tubes in women, and in the urethra (urine canal) in women and men. The bacterium can also grow in the mouth, throat, eyes, and anus. "Having sex" means anal, vaginal, or oral sex. Gonorrhea can still be transmitted via fluids even if a man does not ejaculate. Gonorrhea can also be spread from an untreated mother to her baby during childbirth.

Symptoms: Most women with gonorrhea do not have any symptoms. Even when a woman has symptoms, they are often mild and can be mistaken for a bladder or vaginal infection. The initial symptoms in women can include a painful or burning sensation when urinating, increased vaginal discharge, or vaginal bleeding between periods. Women with gonorrhea are at risk of developing serious complications from the infection, even if symptoms are not present or are mild.

Cure: Gonorrhea can be cured. It's important to take all medication prescribed and to not share medication with anyone. Although medication will stop the infection, it will not repair any permanent damage done by the disease. Drug-resistant strains of gonorrhea are increasing, and successful treatment of gonorrhea is becoming more difficult. If symptoms continue, return to a health care provider to be re-evaluated.

Disease: HIV stands for Human Immunodeficiency Virus. It is the virus that can lead to Acquired Immunodeficiency Syndrome, or AIDS.

Symptoms: The only way to know if you are infected with HIV is to be tested. You cannot rely on symptoms to know whether you have HIV. Many people who are infected with HIV **do not have any symptoms at all** for 10 years or more. Some people who are infected report having flu-like symptoms, often described as "the worst flu ever," two to four weeks after exposure. Symptoms can include: fever, enlarged lymph nodes, sore throat, or rash.

These symptoms can last anywhere from a few days to several weeks. During this time, HIV infection may not show up on a HIV test, but people who have it are highly infectious and can spread the infection to others.

Cure: Unlike some other viruses, the human body cannot get rid of HIV. Once you have HIV, you have it for life. Antiretroviral therapy (ART), however, can dramatically prolong the lives of those infected with HIV and lower the chances of infecting others. It is very important to get tested for HIV early to know if you are infected so medical care and treatment have the greatest effect.

Disease: __Syphilis__ is a sexually transmitted disease (STD) caused by a bacterium. Syphilis can cause long-term complications and/or death if not adequately treated.

Symptoms:

Primary Stage

The appearance of a single sore marks the first (primary) stage of syphilis symptoms, but there may be multiple sores. The sore appears at the location where syphilis entered the body. The sore is usually firm, round, and painless.

Secondary Stage

Skin rashes and/or sores in the mouth, vagina, or anus *(also called mucous membrane lesions)* mark the secondary stage of symptoms. This stage usually starts with a rash on one or more areas of the body. Symptoms can include fever, swollen lymph glands, sore throat, patchy hair loss, headaches, weight loss, muscle aches, and fatigue.

Late and Latent Stages

The latent *(hidden)* stage of syphilis begins when primary and secondary symptoms disappear. Without treatment, an infected person can continue to have syphilis in their body even though there are no signs or symptoms. This latent stage can last for years.

Symptoms of the late stage of syphilis include difficulty coordinating muscle movements, paralysis, numbness, gradual blindness, dementia, and damage to internal organs including the brain, nerves, eyes, heart, blood vessels, liver, bones, and joints. This damage can result in death.

Cure: No home remedy or over-the-counter medicine will cure syphilis, but syphilis is curable with appropriate antibiotics from a physician. Treatment will kill the syphilis bacterium and prevent further damage, but it will not repair damage already done.

For more information on any sexual disease, go to: http://www.cdc.gov

Questions/Reflection

1) **What is the definition of sex?**

    _____

    _____

    _____

2) **How can you become pregnant?**

    _____

    _____

    _____

3) **What are two types of sex?**

    _____

    _____

    _____

4) **Name an STD and its symptoms.**

    _____

    _____

    _____

5) How can you tell if you have HIV?

_____

_____

_____

6) Define one distinction of doing it God's way vs. the world's way.

_____

_____

_____

7) Self-Reflection: Whose way are you following, the world or God's? How are you going to do better?

_____

_____

_____

seven

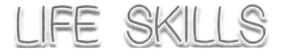

LIFE SKILLS

Give A Man A Fish And You Feed Him For A Day; Show Him How To Catch Fish And You Feed Him For A Lifetime

If you teach someone how to do something instead of doing it for them, they will become self-sufficient.

Let the wise hear and increase in learning, and the one who understands obtain guidance,- *Proverbs 1:5 - ESV*

Dear Divine Daughter,

Becoming a woman requires you to know many things in caring for yourself and eventually others. As I have mentioned before, there are many things that build your worth as a woman (*and as a man - I taught my boys all of these things*) and knowing certain skills is one of them.

Listed below are some life skills on which to build a foundation.

Cleaning – *Cleanliness is next to Godliness*. This is a phrase I used to hear often, but never paid any attention to until I started to care for my own home. God says He likes everything decent and in order and that includes not only our lives, but our homes, as well. My mother is an advocate of having things clean. She started me washing dishes at age nine. Well, I sort of started myself. I begged her to wash dishes thinking it would be fun *(little did I know)*; once she saw I was ready to handle it on my own, it became my regular chore.

As a young woman, having a clean home speaks volumes about your worth. Your home can say you're disorderly, lazy, and unclean or it can say you're neat, clean, and organized like the Proverbs 31 woman. It also determines whether anyone will eat food from your home. As for me, I'm very picky. If I see you have a dirty house, good luck on getting me to eat anything you cook. Many people, including men, feel the same way. I feel if the house is dirty, then the food can't be very clean either. Knowing how to get cleaning solutions and mop, sweep, wipe, and dust every area of your house or room speaks favorably about you as a divine daughter.

No husband wants an unclean wife; he can be a slob all by himself. You have to be an asset to his situation and him to yours. There are so many different cleaning tools and techniques (cleaning, not straightening up) that I can't list them all. Basically, it comes down to if it's dusty, dust it; if it's dirty, clean it; if it's cluttered, organize it. I wish I could show you how it's done; however, there are plenty of tutorials on YouTube and people in your life who are willing to show you. So no excuses!

Laundry – Every young woman needs to know how to wash their own clothes. I started doing my laundry at around age 12. Everyone has a different way of doing it, but generally it simply requires the following:

- Separate your clothes in the following pile types: whites, colors, and delicates (special fabrics – lightweight materials, not *dry clean only*).

- Set the washer according to the type of clothes you are washing, *i.e. whites, colors, etc.*

- Follow the panel instructions to set the washer to the appropriate load size (small, medium or large) and cycle settings

  - When washing whites, set on hot water and normal cycle

  - Colors, set on cold water and normal cycle

  - Delicates, set on either warm or cold water and gentle cycle

- While the wash tub is filling with water, add your detergent *(if it's powder, let it dissolve before adding clothes. Swish it around to help dissolve).*

- Add clothes. If you're using a fabric softener or bleach *(for whites only),* add at the appropriate time stated on the container and\or panel instructions.

- When washer has stopped, take clothes and place in dryer on appropriate temperature for load washed. *Please note: Some delicates may need to be hung or place on a flat surface to air dry, check labels for instructions.*

Cooking – Everybody has to eat and McDonalds, KFC, and Taco Bell won't do, at least, not all the time. You need to learn to cook for yourself and eventually your family, should you have one. This is another worth builder. As a young girl, I had so much fun with my grandmother's cookbook *(while she was at work, of course)* attempting my favorite dishes. Did they all turn out well? Of course not, but at least I tried. When a recipe turned out badly, I figured out what I did wrong so I could do better next time. These little cooking adventures helped me develop my own sense of flavor. Now, I get a recipe and tweak it to my satisfaction by adding my own flavor to it. This came with trial and error, but if I say so myself, I'm a pretty good cook. You can be, too. Just apply yourself.

Nutrition – Being a good cook, as well as a good eater, nutrition wasn't always a big part of my diet or recipes. But as I got older and the pounds started to come, stay, and multiply, I realized it was time to find ways to eat healthy for myself and my family. You will find the foods you put in your body need to add to your health, not take away. Too much of anything is not good, so learn to do things in moderation. Through my years of dieting, I have found the best way to eat healthy and stay fit is to not overindulge in anything. Eat plenty of fruits and vegetables, whole grains, lean proteins, and drink plenty of water. All of these things are good for your overall health, to provide nutrients to feed your body, and to fight off disease and toxins. Fruits and vegetables help to reduce diseases such as heart disease and some cancers. Whole grains and lean proteins help you feel full longer and are used as fuel for your body, unlike white flour, pasta, and rice, which converts to sugar if not burned and turns into fat. Water is the source that keeps all body parts hydrated and moving efficiently. We seldom drink enough, but you should drink at least one ounce for half of your body weight daily (*body weight/2*), or eight 8oz glasses.

It's always a good rule to use moderation when eating sweets or high calorie foods. Your diet should use the 80/20 rule *(that is what I call it)*. Eat healthy 80% of the time, and then you can indulge 20% of the time. You can also make up your own rule depending on where you want to be physically and nutritionally and what works for you.

Fitness – Once you have your diet together, it's time to fine tune your body. Me, myself, and I have never been crazy about exercising. Just recently, I've started a weekly workout routine of Zumba that includes cardio/weight training at least three days a week. I must say, exercise does a body good. I feel well, have a lot more energy, and I look a lot better. You can't beat that.

It doesn't matter if you're not overweight; you still need to work your body and eat healthy.

The sooner you start exercising your body, the better shape it will be in for the long haul, inwardly and outwardly. This is taking care of your temple by literally building muscle to fight off disease that comes and attacks you through poor diet and lack of exercise.

ETIQUETTE

Church

I know we often hear "Come as you are," but there are some things you just shouldn't do while attending church services:

- Dress inappropriately. I know some churches have become more casual with church attire, but nothing should be inappropriate, such as too tight, too short, or too revealing *(respect of appearance).*
- Do not talk or walk around during worship services, especially during altar prayer, the sermon, or altar call.
- Do not text, play games, pass notes, or sleep during worship service. This shows a lack of

respect for the Lord's house and the worship service.

- Do not eat or drink in the sanctuary.
- If you need to leave, do so quietly so you don't interrupt the worship service.
- Do not destroy property or litter on church grounds *(or anywhere else - respect of property)*.

At the Table

First, learn how to set a table:

- A traditional table setting has the napkin and fork to the left of the plate, and the knife (*the blade facing the plate)*, the spoon, and the cup to the right of the plate. The bread and butter plate is optional.

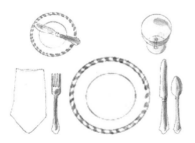

- Formal table settings may include many different forks, knives, and spoons for different courses. Just remember that the utensil farthest from the plate is for the first course, and move inward toward the plate for the later courses.

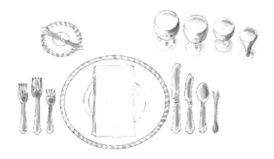

Practice these tips whenever you are at the table:

- Place you napkin on your lap.

- Do not put your elbows on the table.

- If you cannot reach something, politely ask someone else at the table to hand it to you; don't reach over someone to grab it.

- Eat with your silverware, not your hands, unless it is finger food.

- Finish chewing and swallowing before you start talking. Try not to chew with your mouth open.

- Don't play with your food.

- If you sneeze, cough or burp, cover your nose or mouth with your napkin and say, "Excuse me."

- If you notice someone has something in his or her teeth, let them know quietly and do not make a big deal out of it.

- If you spill something, help clean it up.

- Sit tall and interact with the other people at the table.

- If you are at home or a guest at someone else's home, help clear the table once the meal is finished.

- Before you leave the table, make sure the meal is finished and it is appropriate to leave.

Cell Phone

- If you are going somewhere that requires you to be quiet, i.e. church, the movies, school, or the library, set the ringer volume to vibrate or turn it off.

- If it's not appropriate to be on your cell phone, but you are expecting an important call, set the ringer to vibrate and politely excuse yourself when the call comes.

- Never shout into your phone. Not everyone needs to hear your conversation. Be respectful of those around you.

- If you are at home or with your family, set boundaries on when you talk, text, or play games on the phone. If you are at the dinner table, don't answer your cell phone. *Talking, texting, and playing games on your phone takes away valuable time that can be spent with those in your present company.*

- Don't send picture messages or post them on Facebook or any other social website of yourself dressed provocatively, nude, or in a sexual position (*in other words, no sexting – messaging of sexually explicit pictures*).

FINANCE

If you're not a trust fund baby or don't live off your affluent parents, you will need a job to support yourself at some point in time. I have worked since I was 13 years old. I started out babysitting for neighbors until I was old enough to get a "real job." My first real job was working at Braum's Ice Creamery. Words can't express how excited I was to receive my first paycheck, although I thought it should have been much more than it actually was. That's when I found out about FICA and Medicare, in other words the government deductions, which sent a shock to my system. I felt I had worked hard for my money and no one should benefit from my efforts but me, but it is what it is – respect of rules and regulations. Having my own money at a very early age taught me about finance. My mother supplied my needs, but stressed to me that my wants were to be handled by my paycheck, so those new clothes and shoes I wanted would come out of my money. My paycheck was already small which meant I had to learn how to budget to acquire the things I wanted; that was a lot more than I could afford at one time. The options I had at the time were to save up for it, put it in layaway *(the store holds your items for a certain time limit until you pay off the balance)*, or find something cheaper. Needless to say, I've used layaway on many occasions. This taught me to work for what I wanted.

Tithing

As I matured, I learned about tithing, which is giving God one-tenth of my time, talent, and finances through my church. This equips the church to support the church facilities, pastors, staff, missionaries; the poor, the sick and the needy; and to minister to the saved and unsaved in the community.

Why does God requires us to give tithes? Tithing is for <u>our benefit</u>. It teaches us to be unselfish, to put God first, and serves as a reminder that everything belongs to Our Creator. We are only given stewardship (supervision), not ownership, of all that He provides. *Psalms 24:1 – NIV, "The earth is the Lord's, and everything in it, the world, and all who live in it."*

Tithing is an exercise of our faith in God's continued provision. When we step out in faith and give, we learn to trust in God's provision, not money, for our lives by putting Him first through our obedience to His Word.

Tithing is trusting God to meet your needs after you have entrusted Him with the first 10% of your total earnings, regardless of what wants or needs you may have. That equals $10 for every $100 you make *(to whom much is given, much is required)*. God promises to bless you above and beyond for your faith in him. *Luke 6:38, NIV says: "[38] Give and it will be given to you. A good measure, pressed down, shaken together and running over, will be poured into your lap. For with the measure you use, it will be measured to you."* God is not a man that He should lie; He keeps His promises.

When God gives you good measure; it's not always in the form of money. It could come in the form of somebody blessing you with something more valuable than the money you gave.

Short Story: *When my husband and I started to tithe, I was nervous about giving a tenth of our earnings to the church because I feared something would come up and we wouldn't have the money we needed. However, my husband has always had blind faith in God and believed God would do what He says He will do. I try to rationalize things with my carnal (fleshly) mind and what I've come to realize is that a carnal mind can never understand spiritual things. We were going on vacation and before we left, my husband left our tithes/offering with his friend to put in the church offering in our absence. The money he gave him was too much, but he didn't have change. Instead of my husband asking for the change upon our return, he said put it all in. As we were traveling on vacation the muffler went out on our SUV. It was so loud it sounded like a tractor going down the road. My husband pulled over to a shop in a little country town to* *see about getting it repaired. The man examined it and estimated it would cost $1000 to fix. For some reason he said, I wouldn't normally do this except for my friends, but I'll fix it for $30 (God's favor - pressed down, shaken together, running over). That was a $970.00 savings. That's what I call running over. We knew it was God because $30 was the exact change my husband gave over our tithes and offering. God is so good; don't fail to try Him for yourself.*

Credit Cards

Credit cards are useful in the proper context, but as with everything, too much can be a bad thing. Many young people get their first credit card right out of high school and immediately ruin their credit rating. Nothing is free; there are always strings attached. With credit cards that attachment is interest, very high interest *(the cost of borrowing money)*. Credit cards allow you to purchase something you can't afford, so you have to pay even more for it over years to come. I'm not saying credit cards are bad, but temptation and lack of self-control is. We will all encounter credit card temptation and some will fall into the trap of unnecessary debt. In my opinion, the best reason to have a credit card is for emergency purposes only. You'll have to decide what those are, but what they are <u>not</u> is clothes, shoes, jewelry, etc. Other reasons for a credit card:

- To build creditworthiness – you will need to establish good credit to buy a car, house, or rent an apartment. A credit card can help get you started, *if you pay on time, every time.* If not, ***it can destroy your credit*** before you build a credit history. It is much safer to get a pre-paid credit line for this until you get familiarized with the process. That way you can only spend what you have deposited to the account.
- To rent a car or for a hotel stay - you have to provide a credit card to charge against in case of any incidentals. Pay cash for the car or hotel room.
- To purchase something you **<u>need</u>** today that you don't have the cash for, but can pay off

within a billing cycle *(usually a month)* so that no interest charges accrue. The interest charge can be crippling to your pocket book. If you don't pay off your balance by the end of the billing cycle, then you're responsible for the balance plus interest. This is how credit card companies make their money. They're counting on you to charge more than you can afford. Most young people don't realize that the minimum payment requirement is not enough. This just pays on the interest, not the principle amount you charged, which prolongs the time and increases the amount of money owed.

Be very careful not to fall into the credit card trap. It is not free money, but very costly money. Use with caution.

Budgeting

An important element of your finances is learning how to budget your money. A budget is simply a plan of how to allocate and spend your money during a particular timeframe. Budgeting can be a very useful tool when you have to manage household bills. It helps to:

- Avoid spending money on unnecessary items and services.
- Make you aware of your income, how fast it's being spent, and where and to whom it is going.
- Organize your bills so you can decide in advance how your money will work for you.
- See potential money problems in advance and make adjustments before the problem appears.
- Show you how much debt you have incurred, if you can realistically afford it, and if creating the debt is really worth it.
- Avoid wasting money on late fees, penalties, and interests.

Although budgets are very good to have, there is no "one size fits all." Budgets are personalized based on each person's income, spending habits, and obligations. The sooner you create a budget, the better you can keep your finances on track and your spending in check.

In other words:

- Always stay gainfully employed so you have income. If you don't work, you can't buy the things you want and the things you need to survive. *The Bible says in 2 Thessalonians 3:10 – NIV, "The one who is unwilling to work shall not eat."*

- Learn to live within your budget. If you can't buy it right away, save up for it or find a less expensive version. Don't live above your income.

- Always save some money for a rainy day.

- Give some money away, to God first through tithes and offerings, and to other charitable foundations or people in need.

- Pay yourself - you work to pay your expenses, but also to buy the things you want and enjoy.

Questions/Reflections

1) How can you learn to cook?

_____

_____

_____

2) When doing laundry, how do you separate clothes?

_____

_____

_____

3) What is one way to keep your body healthy?

_____

_____

_____

4) What is one reason <u>not</u> to use a credit card?

_____

_____

_____

5) What is tithing?

_____

_____

_____

6) What are some ways you can stay within your budget?

_____

_____

_____

7) Self-Reflection: How do my current life skills measure up? What areas can I improve?

_____

_____

_____

eight

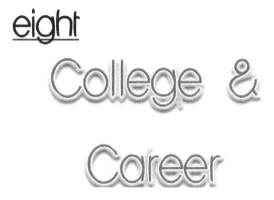

College & Career

"If You Fail To Plan, You Plan To Fail"

"For I know the plans I have for you," declares the LORD, "plans to prosper you and not to harm you, plans to give you a hope and a future." *Jeremiah 29:11 - NIV*

Dear Divine Daughter,

It is so important to have a plan for your life. God's plans are to give you a hope and a future. As a divine daughter, you need to seek Godly wisdom on the direction God has for your life, be it college, trade school, military, the arts, etc.

God created us all to do something and seeking your purpose here on earth should be done with purpose. First and foremost, seek your purpose by asking God what He created you to do.

Knowing your purpose will assist you in following your passion(s).

Short Story: *I started out not really knowing what I wanted to do with my life, but had a long list of things to try. It was a little harder for me because I had my first child at 18, second child at 20, and third child at 23. Needless to say, my choices were limited even with the help of my husband; having children so young made it clear that my main career would be raising my sons and making sure they were provided for. Did I plan this? No. Did I make the best of my situation? Yes. I always planned to go to college and earn a degree. After having my children, that dream was delayed. I couldn't go when I had planned,* ***but God's*** *future for me allowed me to go. I graduated Cum Laude in 2007, from LeTourneau University, as a business major. Even though my plans were delayed, they were* *not denied. The key is I had a plan and never gave up on it. However, there is one thing I wish I had done earlier: Simply asked God, "What is my purpose for being here?" It would have saved a lot of time and effort trying to figure things out on my own and saved years of guess work. Time waits for no one. Ask God what your purpose is and do all you can, while you can. No excuses.*

Determining your life path has a lot to do with researching and exploring things that interest you; finding your passion and purpose. Your passion is what you love to do; what gets you motivated. Your purpose is to operate in the fullness of which you were created. Let your spirit guide you. God has put so many unique gifts inside you; you need to explore what He purposed for your life. Many times, we are unaware of the career paths that are available to us because we don't research what lines up with our passion and purpose. With the internet, it's much easier than it once was to research career options; the world is literally at your fingertips. I have always heard that if you make a career out of your passion you never work a day in your life. Tap into what you're passionate about and align it with a career that will stimulate you mentally, spiritually, and financially. Some things you are passionate about might not be as profitable as other career choices, but money isn't everything. If you don't know that now, you'll find out one day – hopefully. Peace of mind and helping others can be much more rewarding. However, you do need to make enough to support yourself and eventually your family. Just don't determine your career by money alone. Make sure it's something you enjoy doing since it will consume many hours of your day.

> **"If You Make a Career Out Of Your Passion**
> **You Never Work a Day in Your Life"**

Reflect on your purpose and your passion, align it with a career that interests you, and work your plan in achieving the criteria you need to get into the career field that you desire.

Questions you should ask yourself:

1. What is my purpose/passion?

2. How can I make it profitable?

3. What requirements do I need to meet?

Examples:

Passion – Styling Hair

Career – Hair Stylist, Instructor, Salon Owner

Criteria – Cosmetology School

Passion/Purpose– Teaching

Career – Teacher/Professor

Criteria – College –Educational Degree(s)

Passion – Website/Print Publications

Career – Graphic Design Artist

Criteria – College/Trade School

Passion – Debating

Career – Lawyer/Politician

Criteria – College – Law School

Passion/Purpose – Preaching the Word of God

Career – Pastor/Preacher/Evangelist

Criteria – College – Seminary School

Passion – Math

Career – Accountant/Financial Advisor

Criteria – College – Business/Accounting

Passion – Science/Prosthetics

Career – Biomedical Engineer

Criteria – College – Medical School

It's not difficult to pick a career based on your passion or purpose, that is, if you know what your passion or purpose is, but it's also not easy to go into a career without first getting an education. That part of the process will take dedication, time, and money that you and your parents may not have. If you dedicate the time to obtain an education to have a career, there are many avenues you can take to get funding. The most common methods, in order of preference, are as follows:

- **Scholarships** – Scholarships are free money usually given on **merit-basis** *(academic or athletic achievement, extracurricular or artistic performance)*. There are various scholarships for all types of things, i.e. career fields, ethnicity, church affiliation, etc., that are waiting on qualified candidates to apply for them, but many students don't take the time to apply. Speak to your counselor and/or look them up on the internet. Make sure to submit your application before the deadline and beware of any scams.

- **Grants** – Grants are free money often given on a **need-basis.** After submitting your Free Application for Federal Student Aid, or FAFSA, you are notified if you qualify for any state or federal grants and the amount(s) as well as any financial aid you might qualify for in the form of loans (see Student Loans). You can also apply for grants through the following: Colleges and Universities, Public and Private Organizations, and Professional Associations.

- **Community College** – If you didn't apply or don't qualify for scholarships or grants, you can save money on the first two years of college by living at home and attending a community college to take your general *(basic)* education classes *(making excellent grades, of course)*, then transfer to a university to finish your core classes. This will allow you to get acclimated to college life, save money on room and board, and classes without spending a lot of money out of pocket or borrowing.

- **Student Loans** – These are loans that are given out by the government and private lenders. They rarely go away without full repayment of the loan along with accrued interest. You may be able to get credit for nonprofit organization work, but most likely you will pay off the principal and interest over a lifetime. *Make this your absolute last solution to pay college tuition.*

DRESSING FOR SUCCESS

When searching for a career, you always want to dress for success by making sure you are well groomed and have a polished look. This includes:

- Wearing clothing that is clean, wrinkle free, and comfortable.

- Wearing clothing that is respectable; not too short, not too tight *(doesn't require continuous adjustment when sitting, standing, or walking),* and not too loud in color.

- Styling your hair so that it's not too dramatic in color or style.

- Wearing small to medium sized earrings (*one pair will suffice*) and no flashy jewelry.

- Wearing closed-toe shoes; no house shoes, flip-flops, or slide-ons.

- Wearing natural looking make-up; nothing too dramatic or over the top.

- Wearing natural looking nails with a clear or neutral polish; don't wear long, flashy, brightly colored nails.

- Wearing softly scented perfume or body oil that's not overpowering.

- Wearing your most beautiful smile and <u>no</u> chewing gum.

Tattoos and Piercings

It's becoming a rite of passage to get tattoos and piercings, but what young people don't think about before they get tattoos and piercing is how it will affect their career choices. Depending on what type of career you choose, getting tattoos and piercings that are visible can limit your chances of a lucrative career in several fields, including the military. Just because it's something that everyone is doing doesn't mean it is right for you. Don't put limits on yourself by trying to follow a fad or trend. Having a plan for your life includes not putting hindrances on your options.

Questions/Reflection

1) How do you find your purpose in life?

_____

_____

_____

2) How do you turn your passion into a career?

_____

_____

_____

3) What are some examples of professions that align with your passion?

_____

_____

_____

4) How do you get funding for your education?

_____

_____

_____

5) How do you make sure you are dressing for success?

_____

_____

_____

6) What are some hindrances you can put on your choices for careers?

_____

_____

_____

7) Self-Reflection: What is my purpose and/or passion? What steps am I going to take to make a career out of my purpose/passion?

_____

_____

_____

nine

YOUR

SALVATION

"Without God <u>YOU</u> Can Do Nothing"

"For God so loved the world that he gave his one and only Son, that whoever believes in him shall not perish but have eternal life." *John 3:16 - NIV*

Dear Divine Daughter,

To become a "Daughter of Divine Destiny" your first step is to become a believer in the Trinity; God, the Father, Jesus, the Son, and the Holy Spirit that dwells in you upon your acceptance of Jesus as your Savior. It is necessary for you to know God before you can apply any of the principles in this book to your life.

In **Philippians 4:13 – KJV, it states: "I can do all things through Christ who strengtheneth me."** If you don't know God, then it will be impossible for your destiny to be divine, heavenly, or Godly. In order to put the characteristics in this book into action, you first have to believe in God and want to live according to **His Will and His Purpose for your life**.

We all will be presented an opportunity to accept Jesus as our Savior; some will wait until they're ready *(whenever and whatever that means)* and some will accept Jesus with open arms right away. I was one who wanted to wait because I believed accepting Jesus as my Savior meant living a life that would be boring and full of things I wanted to do but couldn't. I couldn't wait to get out of my mother's house to have the freedom to do what I wanted to do. I thought accepting Jesus meant putting even more constraints on my life that I was trying to get rid of. So I waited to develop a relationship with God and lived my life by my rules and regulations when I got out on my own. It worked for a while; I was happy doing what I wanted to do, when I wanted to do it, not having anyone to tell me otherwise. You see, I grew up going to church all day every Sunday, literally from sunup to sundown. I remember when we didn't have a car and my mother, my brothers, and I walked to church. Church was in my system; it was a part of my foundation. I remember not being able to wear pants to church and getting criticized when I colored my hair or wore makeup. Needless to say, I didn't like the church traditions. When I had my chance to have a say in my life after I left my mother's house, I didn't go to church for several years. When I did go it was for special occasions; a funeral or whenever I felt like going. It was after having children that I realized they needed a moral foundation, so I started going to church more frequently to give them that foundation. It wasn't until something tragic happened that I realized it was time to turn things around.

Short Story: It was year 1994 when tragedy struck our family. My uncle, Abner Lewis

Campbell, whom we called Uncle Ab, was the lively uncle of our family. He died in a tragic car accident; he was only 39 years old. This same accident also injured another uncle who is only two years older than I am. The ultimate tragedy of this event wasn't Uncle Ab's death, but the fact that we didn't know if Uncle Ab had accepted Jesus as his Lord and Savior; he also waited. We will never know if he ever got it right between himself and the Lord. In November of 1994, my grandfather, the Elder Leonard Campbell, preached my Uncle Ab's eulogy. In December of that same year, my grandfather died a day after Uncle Ab's 40th birthday, December 27th. It was at this time I realized time waits for no one, no matter how young or old you are. If you don't get your business straight with God while you still have breath in your body, you can surely pass away without being saved, or anyone knowing if you were saved or not.

In December of 1994, I confessed with my mouth to my church family that I accepted Jesus as my Lord and Savior, that I truly believed in my heart that He died and rose on the third day morning, and is alive, sitting on the right hand side of God the Father, making intercession *(intervention)* on behalf of all believers. I was 23 years old; still young, but now assured of my salvation. You can go to church your whole life because your family makes you or takes you, but there will come a time when you have to make it personal and know that you know, that you know He is Lord and **you accept Him as Lord of your life**. I can honestly say I missed nothing of the life I wanted to live according to my will and each day with Jesus is sweeter than the day before because He brings true meaning to my purpose for being. Since I have established a relationship with God, he speaks to my spirit, guiding me to live according to His Will and His Purpose for my life. I must say it's far from boring and I can do the things I like to do; now I just do them decent and in order or not at all. If I ever find myself getting out of the Will of God, He convicts my spirit to get me back on the right path.

> "I know my redeemer lives; I spoke with him this morning." –
> Nicole C. Mullen

My first question for you is **Do you accept God as your Lord and Savior Jesus Christ?** By answering **YES**, you are saying you believe the following:

We are all sinners - You are a sinner – you do wrong things:

Romans 3:10 - NIV – As it is written: "There is no one righteous, not even one; - No one is without sin, we all do wrong things.

Romans 3:23 - NIV – for all have sinned and fall short of the glory of God, - We all sin daily and fall short of being in right standing with God.

Sin's Punishment - Your punishment for being a sinner:

Romans 5:12 - NIV – Therefore, just as sin entered the world through one man (Adam), and death through sin, and in this way death came to all people, because all sinned Adam was the first man to commit sin, by his disobedience in the Garden of Eden by eating the fruit from the tree of knowledge, which God had forbidden. His punishment for eating the fruit was death among other things. Since we are all descendants of Adam, we are a part of a generational curse where we are all sentenced to death. *Read Genesis 3 in its entirety.*

Jesus Paid for Our Punishment - You don't have to take your punishment; Jesus already took it for you:

Romans 5:8 - NIV – But God demonstrates His own love towards us in this: While we were still sinners, Christ died for us. Jesus' blood that he shed on the cross paid for our punishment. Jesus served as the sacrificial lamb for all of our sins and died on the cross so that we may have eternal life.

Romans 6:23 - NIV – For the wages of sin is death, but the gift of God is eternal life in Christ Jesus our Lord. We were all under a curse until God gave us the gift of life through His son, Jesus Christ.

We Have Salvation through our Faith - By believing in God, you will have eternal life:

Romans 10:9-10 - NIV – [9] **If you declare** *(confess)* **with your mouth, "Jesus is Lord," and believe in your heart that God raised him from the dead, you will be saved.** [10] **For it is with your heart that you believe and are justified, and it is with your mouth that you profess your faith and are saved.** This confession is very important because this is your formal, spiritual acceptance of Jesus Christ as your Lord and Savior. There's no getting around it because God knows your heart.

Romans 10:13 - NIV – **for, "Everyone who calls on the name of the Lord will be saved."** Everyone who accepts Jesus as their personal Savior will be saved. Jesus is a gift; you don't have to pay for it, you don't have to work for it, you just have to accept Him like you would a gift.

Romans 10:17 - NIV – **Consequently, faith comes from hearing the message, and the message is heard through the Word about Christ.** Your faith in God comes by hearing the

Word of God (the Bible) and applying the principles to your life, which builds your trust and belief in God.

If you have confessed with your mouth and you truly believe in your heart that God raised Jesus from the dead, you are now saved and are welcomed into the family of Jesus Christ.

You need to connect and get involved with a bible-based church so you can grow in faith by hearing and studying the Word of God, to live a life pleasing unto God. You also need to establish a personal relationship with God by communicating with Him on a daily basis through meditating on His Word and prayer *(a spoken or unspoken address to God, to express praise, thanksgiving, confession, or a request for something such as help or for someone's well-being)*. The first prayer I learned was the "Lord's Prayer" found in;

Matthew 6:9-13 – KJV:

[9] After this manner therefore pray ye: Our Father which art in heaven, Hallowed be thy name.

[10] Thy kingdom come, Thy will be done in earth, as it is in heaven.

[11] Give us this day our daily bread.

[12] And forgive us our debts, as we forgive our debtors.

[13] And lead us not into temptation, but deliver us from evil: For thine is the kingdom, and the power, and the glory, forever.

In Jesus' name, Amen.

You should always close your prayers with "In Jesus' Name." It puts a stamp on your prayers to deliver them to God. Remember, Jesus is sitting on the right-hand side of God reminding Him that your sins are covered by His blood.

**Let God's Word Be Your Moral Compass –
What You Live By!**

ten

Words of
Wisdom

When You Know Better, You Should Do Better...

Blessed are those who find wisdom, those who gain understanding, *Proverbs 3:13 - NIV*

Finally, *Daughters of Divine Destiny*, there are some things you need to know to make life worth living a little easier. Listed are a few nuggets of wisdom to encourage you on your journey:

Listen to Learn and Learn to Listen to Constructive Criticism – To have an advantage in life, you need to be able to learn from other people's mistakes and successes. As well as, listen to constructive criticism (useful critique) of yourself. It will get you farther in life with fewer mishaps.

Tap Into Your Purpose/Passion – We all have a purpose and a passion to do something. You might not know what it is or have yet to tap into it; however, you need to be about something other than yourself or the next party that's jumping. An idle mind is the devil's workshop. Pray and ask God to show you your purpose in life; what he created you for. In the meantime, try different things to see if you like them. If you are a mother, develop a passion to raise intelligent, God-fearing, productive children of society.

You Have To Do What You Have To Do In Order To Do What You Want To Do – Anything in life worth having requires work. Nothing is just handed to you. *"To whom much is given, much is required."* You can be your own worst enemy with procrastination, lack of discipline, laziness, and not having enough or the right education. Also, remember that you may fail at times, but failure is not final if you get back up. If you never try, you have already failed.

Love Yourself – Self validation will allow you to love yourself respectfully when you feel no one else does. Loving yourself will allow you to not let others treat you disrespectfully or harm you and yours. It all begins and ends with self. Take care of yourself and love yourself first, then you're able to take care of everybody else.

Just because you have a strong opinion about something doesn't mean you are right. Go to the Word and find what God says about it.

Heartbreak is not the end of the world; learn from it and move on. Being single is not always a bad thing.

Quit Putting the Cart Before the Horse; doing things backwards. Remember that God says He wants things decent and in order.

Why buy the cow, when the milk is free? Don't give him the benefits of a husband when he not asking you to be his wife.

Don't have more children than you can take care of on your own, because you just might have to care for them all by yourself.

Be careful who you let watch your children; not everyone is qualified.

Live a life that you and your children will be proud of.

Your worth doesn't decrease based on someone's inability to see your value.

If you spend time regretting the past, you lose the present and risk the future.

The choices you make today, will be the choices you have to live with tomorrow.

Let your dreams be bigger than your fears and your actions louder than your words. Make your time count!

Proverbs 3:5-6 – KJV, *[5] Trust in the LORD with all thine heart; and lean not unto thine own understanding.[6] In all thy ways acknowledge him, and he shall direct thy paths.*

Encouragement – This, Too, Shall Pass

In life, we are destined to go through some trials and tribulations no matter who we are or how good we have been, no matter what we might get caught up in or bring on ourselves. We live in a world where trouble and affliction have no respect of a person and will come at you in your most vulnerable time, but if you have your life grounded in the Word of God you can weather those storms, knowing God has His hands on you and that This, Too, Shall Pass. I want you to know that nothing is too hard for God, no matter how tough or dire the situation may look. There is always joy in the morning, because trouble doesn't last always. You have to be strong in the Word of God, to know you can make it and stand no matter what may come your way. This world is only temporary and only what you do for Christ will last. You have to know that your hopes and dreams should be built on nothing less than the eternal things of God. Remember, *Matthew 6:33-KJV," 33 but seek ye first the kingdom of God, and his righteousness; and all these things shall be added unto you."* If you put God first,

He will fight your battles for you. Get into His Word so that when the world comes at you, you can be prepared to say **God's Got It and This, Too, Shall Pass**.

Divine Daughters,

I want you to know that you are not alone and the saints of the Lord are all praying for your strength and growth in the Lord. If you ever need to talk, express your feelings, want to share a praise report or have a question and need Godly wisdom, go to: **divine-daughters.com** *and post a question or comment. You can remain anonymous and we will be sure to respond. God bless you and we love you!*

References

- http://www.loveisrespect.org

- http://women.webmd.com

- More Than a Hero: Muhammad Ali's Life Lessons through His Daughter's Eyes

- http://afropuffsandponytails.com

- http://www.pamf.org/preteen/growingup/etiqu ette.html#At the Table

- http://www.emilypost.com/table-manners/71-table-setting-guides

- http://chealth.canoe.ca/channel_section_deta ils.asp?text_id=5649&channel_id=7&relation_ id=24636

- http://opensourceecology.org/wiki/7_Areas_o f_Respect

- www.cdc.gov

- My Redeemer Lives; Nicole C. Mullen

- http://www.drugabuse.gov/drugs-abuse

Scripture References

1 Corinthians 6:19 (NIV)

1 Corinthians 6:18-20 (NIV)

1 Corinthians 7:2 (NIV)

1 Corinthians 14:40 (KJV

1 Thessalonians 3:10 (NIV)

Genesis 2:24 (KJV)

Genesis 3 (NIV)

Hosea 4:6 (NIV)

Jeremiah 29:11 (NIV)

John 3:16 (NIV)

John 10:10 (NIV)

Luke 6:38 (NIV)

Matthew 6:33 (NIV)

Matthew 7:12 (NIV)

Philippians 4:13 (KJV)

Proverbs 1:5 (ESV)

Proverbs 3:5-6 (KJV)

Proverbs 4:23 (NIV)

Proverbs 18:24 (NLT)

Proverbs 22:6 (KJV)

Proverbs 29:11 (NIV)

Proverbs 31:10-31 (NIV)

Psalms 24:1 (NIV)

Psalms 139:13-14 (NIV)

Romans 3:10 (NIV)

Romans 3:23 (NIV)

Romans 5:8 (NIV)

Romans 5:12 (NIV)

Romans 6:23 (NIV)

Romans 8:28 (NIV)

Romans 10:9-10 (NIV)

Romans 10:13 (NIV)

Romans 10:17 (NIV)

Romans 12:1 (KJV)

Romans 12:2 (ESV)

Titus 2:3-5 (NIV)

CPSIA information can be obtained at www.ICGtesting.com
Printed in the USA
LVOW01s0518110414

381311LV00002B/2/P